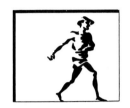

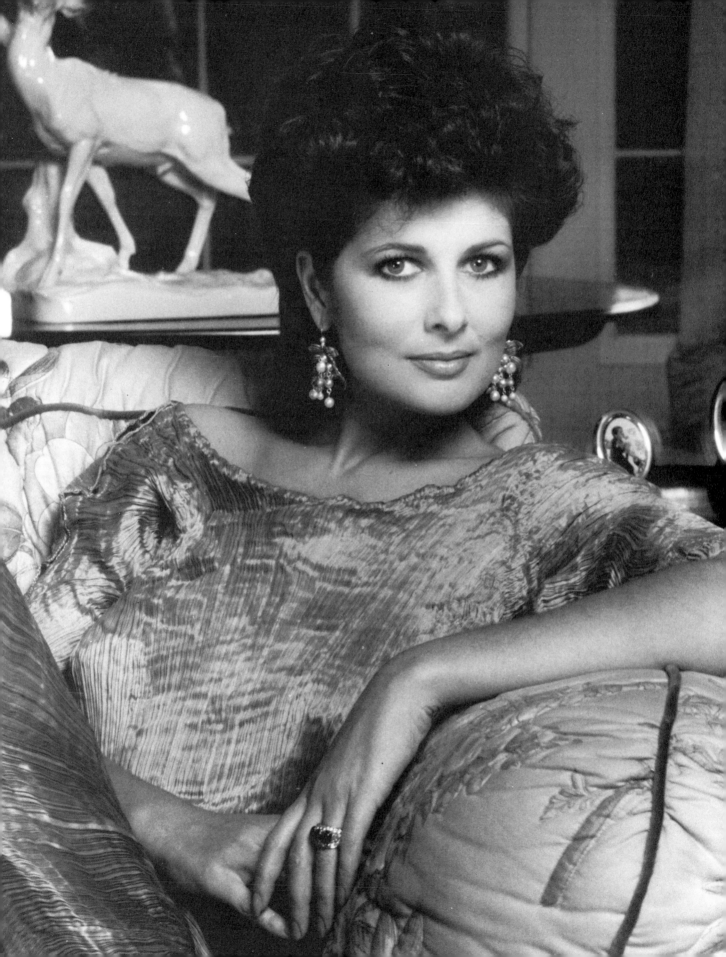

CRISTINA FERRARE

Style

HOW TO HAVE IT IN EVERY PART OF YOUR LIFE

BY

Cristina Ferrare DeLorean

AND *Sherry Suib Cohen*

PHOTOGRAPHS BY ROGER PRIGENT

SIMON AND SCHUSTER · NEW YORK

Published by Simon and Schuster
A Division of Simon & Schuster, Inc.
Simon & Schuster Building
Rockefeller Center
1230 Avenue of the Americas
New York, New York 10020
SIMON AND SCHUSTER and colophon are registered trademarks of Simon & Schuster, Inc.

Designed by Elizabeth Woll

Manufactured in the United States of America
Printed and bound by The Murray Printing Co, Forge Village, Mass.

10   9   8   7   6   5   4   3   2   1

Library of Congress Cataloging in Publication Data
DeLorean, Cristina Ferrare.
   Style.

   1. Beauty, Personal.   2. Women—Health and hygiene.
3. Fashion.   4. Entertaining.   I. Cohen, Sherry Suib.
II. Title.
RA778.D27   1984   646.7′042   84-1380
ISBN 0-671-46849-9

All photographs (except where otherwise noted) © 1983 Roger Prigent.
Hair and makeup (unless otherwise noted) by James Weis.
Drawings by Lamont O'Neal.

DEDICATION

To Al, my pal,
for friendship above and beyond
the call of duty

———————

Acknowledgments

To *my mother and father* for a happy childhood filled with love, closeness, tradition, and humor, for a feeling of self-worth—all of which are reflected in my adult life.

To *Zachary* and *Kathryn* for making me realize that children are not a sacrifice but a privilege.

To *Cindy Brady* for her loyalty and great friendship. My life would not be as organized or secure without her. She is the greatest example of what to aspire to be as a person.

To *Eileen Fairchild*, my best friend, for making me laugh even when I didn't want to —for being there.

To *Maur Dubin* for teaching me about style—often in a maddening way, but always effectively.

To *Sherry Suib Cohen* for her endless patience and for making me feel I really had something to say. I have a new friend.

To *Roger Prigent*. He is responsible for most of the photographs in this book. I don't think I could have worked with anyone else on this project. He has been so patient and loving. I think the photographs reflect that. *Je te remercie, mon cher ami.*

To *Albert Capraro* and *Carmine Porcelli* for their generosity and friendship.

To *Nina Blanchard*. As of the publishing of this book, I am entering my twentieth year as a model. I have had a glorious and successful career. Nina was my first agent, and still is. She saw me through all my ups and downs. Times of great joy and times of sadness. She is my second mother. I can't quite put into words how much she means to me, but I know she feels it.

To *Gary Pudney*. Gary was the first person I called that fateful night in October (John's arrest). He has always been there for me no matter what kind of trouble I was in. I love this man. His compassion, wit and humor helped me in situations I thought I would never be able to get through.

To *Arthur Gregory*, my manager. I don't think anyone I know has been put through more grief because of me. His love and loyalty is unlimited. We are partners for life. I can't wait to start paying his commission!!!

To *Eileen* and *Jerry Ford.* To be a Ford model is the optimum. To have Eileen and Jerry as friends is another matter altogether. All their girls are special, but the love the three of us have for one another is unique. You know at all times where you stand with Eileen, and I'm proud that I stand at the top of her list. These are people of integrity, honor and great Style. I've always been proud to be a Ford model.

To *Deborah Szekely,* founder of the Golden Door spa. There isn't any one individual who has influenced my life as profoundly as Deborah. A truly outstanding person. I have so much respect and regard for everything this remarkable woman has accomplished. She has changed my way of thinking about myself and my attitude toward life in general.

To the "F" team (*The Face Team*): *Francesco, Way & Suga. Francesco Scavullo,* who gave me my first *big* break. He put me on the cover of *Cosmopolitan* and then followed it up with eight pages in *Vogue.* He has been a wonderful friend. Whenever someone asks me who I would prefer to shoot the picture, it is always, *Scavullo!!!* No one has ever photographed me the way he has.

Way Bandy. He has brought this visage through many stages and managed to create an incomparable illusion each time. He is a true artist and a lovely person. Some of the happiest and craziest moments of my life have been sharing secrets and singing opera in the dressing room, often to the dismay of the clients.

Suga. For his gentle spirit, friendship, compassion and love. Whenever I needed a favor he was always there to help me. I have been so fortunate to have had the opportunity to work with and get to know people like this. Thank you, Suga, and Happy Birthday!

To *God.* For an incredible life and career. For all the blessings bestowed on me. For all the people who have come into and out of my life. For loving me.

To *John,* my life . . .

Cristina Ferrare DeLorean

Contents

Preface

STYLE, in the real world, is not a *Harper's Bazaar* cover. I've been on many covers and I also live in the real world—and believe me, there's a difference.

Certainly the glamorous life of a fashion model, the top money, the travel with famous and fascinating company, the fun of being recognized and loved all over the world can get to be very familiar after a while. It may feel like the real world. But it's not. The real world is waking up in the morning, making breakfast for your family, helping the kids with homework. The real world is your face in the mirror when you wake up—before the makeup and the million-dollar outfits. And the real world can be disaster also. There's never disaster in a fashion magazine.

It hit my life and family when my husband was involved in a drug charge that rocked the headlines in every newspaper. We knew he was innocent, but the world knew only what it read, and an ugly backlash from the press and uninformed public opinion fell on us like a ton of bricks. All the good looks, money, and popularity couldn't help me. All the fabled friends were suddenly gone. It's hard to think about style when your husband is threatened. The world no longer reads like a glossy magazine.

But I am convinced that there is something that will turn it all around again —is already turning it around—and that something is attitude. You'll read that word a lot in this book. It's my personal solution to almost everything. There's no question in my mind that a woman who has the right outlook, who believes she has the power to change things around, will. Despite lack of money or beauty, despite even personal disaster, she can move through her days with style—carry on with assurance and grace.

Being stylish if you're Princess Diana is not too difficult. In the real world, however, it's not always sunny; you're not always thin, beautiful, rich, or lucky in love. Sometimes you don't fit into that size eight, and, what's more, you're relieved if the size twelve goes over your hips. Sometimes you lose all your money, your child needs a dermatologist, your prince is dethroned.

In the princess's world, money problems are not major, I'd suspect, but in the real world, you might have to make do with something less than a princess's fortune. Nevertheless, your life can be lived with flair and color. You can dress and entertain and work with genuine style. When you have the right attitude, you don't have to depend on money or luck because you look at the world in an original way. You pay attention to beauty in all things. You have confidence. And you understand that you have a responsibility to celebrate life and yourself and all that you can become.

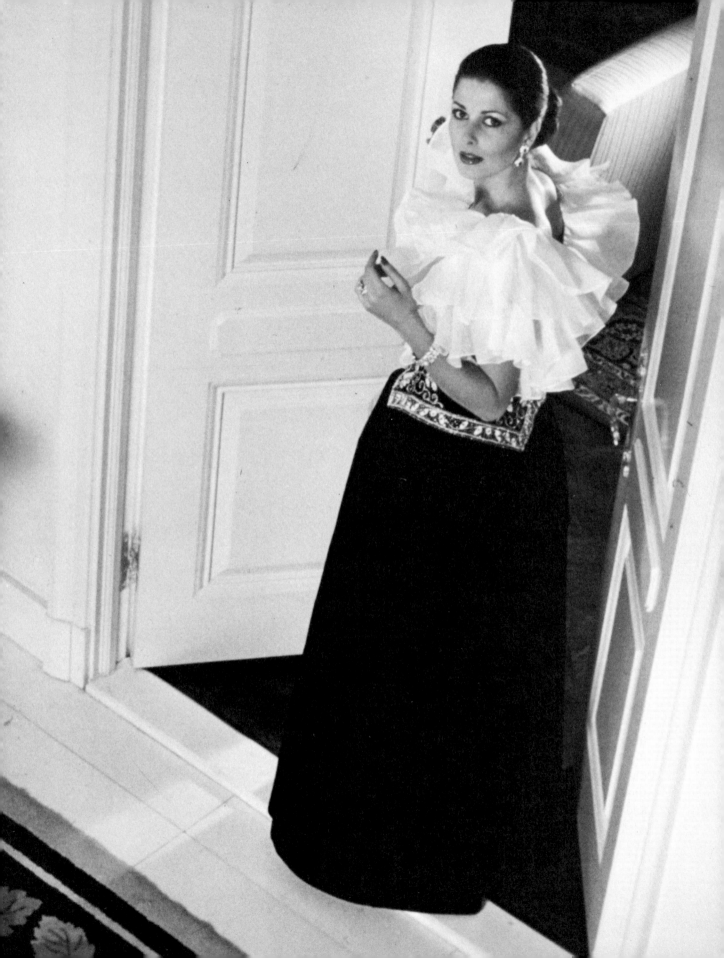

Chapter 1

DRESSING WITH STYLE

*P*ROBABLY the first thing that comes to mind with the word *style* is clothing.

A woman with style and presence understands that high fashion is there to enhance, delight the eye, create a mood, and *not* to disguise one's true self. She doesn't wear someone else's "look," she isn't a wreck about making choices, and she has such a sense of her own clothing integrity that she doesn't need constant outside reassurance.

She's a "natural"—but make no mistake: She does not rely on natural beauty of face or form to dictate her stunning look. She has learned how to create it herself. Anyone can have high style. Really. It doesn't matter what you look like or how many big bucks you have rattling around in your pocket. The only thing that does matter is your ability to express your uniqueness through exciting and chic clothing. Face it: You're never going to look exactly like Cheryl Tiegs or Christie Brinkley. I'm never going to have Christie Brinkley's hips. But each of us is capable of consummate style, for style is, after all, simply an illusion. It's the message our clothes sing out. When I look at Diana Vreeland, Jackie Kennedy Onassis, or Lena Horne, I do *not* think . . .

- over forty
- wrinkles
- imperfect features
- insecure

In fact, the total image that hits my mind's eye is . . .

- classy
- chic
- confident
- STYLE

The individual truths—the age, wrinkles, or imperfections—are virtually hidden in the effect of the whole illusion.

Above all things, the way we dress is positively lyrical, as it tells people about our brand of style—or nonstyle. Clothing conveys messages, double messages, innuendoes, and sometimes lies about one's job, ethnic characteristics, sexual preferences, moods, character, and personality.

"My clothes keep my various selves buttoned up together," wrote the essayist Logan Pearsall Smith, "and enable [them] to pass themselves off as one person."

Think of it this way: The colors, accessories, and fashion we choose define us more easily than a written biographical sketch. Some of the things clothing can say are:

- I'm the new woman at the top.
- I'm very rich.
- I'm sexually available.
- I'm just a scared little incompetent person.
- I'm a blazing intellectual.
- I'm Super-Mom (Super-Model, Super-Lawyer, Super-Depressed, Super-Jock, and so on).
- I'm doomed to fail.
- Trust me—I cannot fail.

Sometimes, accidentally, the messages you give off with clothing are absolutely inaccurate in the expression of *you*. Say you're really terribly shy and withdrawn. Say your cousin lends you her plunging-neckline sheath (the one with the bangles) for your new, blind date. "It's *you!*" she exclaims with exultation. But it isn't you at all, and the blind date's first impression of you is absolutely inaccurate—thanks to your clothing.

Sometimes you *want* to give a clothing message that's not the right message. If you want to send out vibes that you're hale and hearty and a real sports jock, wear a tennis dress or a warm-up suit; even if you haven't held a tennis racquet in twenty years, you'll give off a Chrissie Evert Lloyd persona. Want them to think you're a business executive when you're really a belly dancer? Wear a three-piece gray tweed suit and pumps. You've got the lie made.

The funny thing is, even if people know better, the way you dress at a given moment can sway them. The boy next door, with whom you grew up, can be convinced you mean *business* business in a tweed suit. Clothing, like magic and makeup, creates illusions. Even if you're not rich or famous, you can look it. Even if you're not the boss, you can be a person of great authority if your tailored suit says, "I'm in charge here." On the other hand, you can be, say, the staunchest feminist in the world, a regular Gloria Steinem in character, and if your clothes read baby doll, frilly, pink-y—who's going to believe it? Clothes talk. They may not say what you want them to say about you. They may not even tell the truth at all. That's why it's important for you to face up to your dress style—which has something to do with what's currently fashionable but a lot more to do with what looks good on you and what you really want to say about yourself. Gaucho pants or miniskirts may be the hottest items, but you'll look like a powerless fool if you wear them to work at the brokerage house. Don't misunderstand my use of the word *power*, either. A powerhouse doesn't have to be a woman who is only interested in on-the-job power in the working arena. You can be a powerhouse at the cocktail party, in the bedroom, or in the kitchen as well. You simply have to dress the part you play—wherever you play it. That's fashion in the real world—not on the cover of *Vogue*.

The Biggest Mistakes in Power Dressing

NOT SENSING WHICH WAY THE WIND BLOWS. Will your daughter's friends relate to a mother who wears her hair in ribbon-tied bunches, her skirt above her knees, her anklet-clad feet in saddle shoes? Or will they think she's pushing too hard to look *their* age, to look like their pal instead of their pal's mother? No wonder your daughter acted so surly after the terrific party you threw for her. She wasn't grateful at all, and you couldn't put your finger on the reason why.

I'll tell you why: She was unhappy because you looked inappropriate and that embarrassed her. You lost some good mother power credits even if *you* think you looked pretty adorable in saddle shoes. Even if you *did* look adorable. Dressing well has a lot to do with *who's* seeing your outfits. Adorable stops at a certain age—how about ten?

FEAR OF FASHION. Oh, I know it's popular to say you should only be concerned with your own style, not with the fashion magazines of the world. But that's really too simplistic to have much truth. Peasant dresses look inappropriate at a time when *no one's* wearing peasant dresses except potato farmers in Russia. You have to be somewhat conscious of "what's in." And it's no good to stick to the basic blacks and dreary creams that are always in because that labels you as unimaginative. But don't wear whatever *they* say: Wear what looks good *and* what is also fashionable. Only Margaret Meads can ignore fashion altogether; and that's because women like that are making the "I-don't-care-about-clothes-at-all" statement. That's okay if you're a Margaret Mead. Everybody else, watch out. The best way to cure a fear of fashion is to experiment with a few easy changes in your "comfortable" look. Don't be afraid of making mistakes—take a chance on style.

NOT UNDERSTANDING WHAT TRUE STYLE IS. Style is a certain open-mindedness—a way of looking at clothes that's just a little bit different. A way of *surprising* yourself and others with an unusual color, an unexpected material—a white linen blouse, for instance, with a velvet jacket. It's what makes Mary Tyler Moore look absolutely glamorous in a white taffeta jumpsuit, Jane Fonda exciting in a fringed copper leather jacket, suede jeans, and a felt cowboy hat, and Jessica Tandy stunning in a simple blouse and skirt. True style always involves art. Art can be the way a hat shades the eyes, adding mystery to a face. Oscar Wilde once said that he read the following words in a French magazine under the drawing of a bonnet: "With this style, the mouth is worn slightly open." With true individual style, the mouth can be worn open—or closed. The clothes make their own statement.

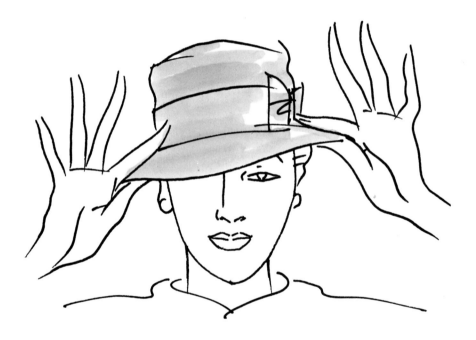

DRESSING FOR THE OCCASION. It's always a *huge* mistake to dress for occasions. One should, instead, dress for people and the way your image will hit them. At any truly fashionable party, for instance, you might see women dressed in many types of attire—terrific pants, cocktail dresses, skirts and silk shirts, tweed suits, and maybe even culottes—with *all* looking perfectly correct and comfortable. Good taste and style are dictated by fabric and design. And the tenor of the times says that if you understand how to choose fabric and design, the *kinds* of outfits you choose (within reason) will always be appropriate. That means that a stunning pantsuit is acceptable in the office today when only a dress would have done fifteen years ago. Naturally, you don't wear cleavage cut down to *here* at the office no matter how tasteful the fabric, but you can be reasonably inventive.

MIXED-UP COMBOS THAT DON'T WORK
- Slinky, strappy shoes with tailored slacks
- A great silk dress—under a bomber jacket
- A velvet blazer—over a summer cotton skirt
- Dark, smoky stockings—with white shoes

You can spend a fortune on clothes, but if you combine them foolishly, you might as well shop in any old Bargain Basement.

ADORABLE-CUTESY. Bows in the hair after age twenty-five, or even at the waist, make you look gift-wrapped and not Sweet Sixteen at all. You have to throw out the fashion look you enjoyed as a teenager just as you have to reevaluate your makeup and hair if you're still wearing doe eyes and bangs.

MAKING TOO MUCH OF A GOOD THING. One good thing is super. Wearing the good thing in every incarnation possible makes it gauche. A fantastic leather belt is a fashion plus. The belt, plus leather pants, a leather jacket, leather handbag, and leather headband yell out, "I Am a Member of a Motorcycle Gang!" A hand-knit sweater is gorgeous. The sweater plus a hand-knit skirt, a hand-painted blouse, and handmade jewelry yell out, "Homemade!"

TYPECASTING. You can typecast yourself in the look you like—and that's your personal style—but you should not always wear the same thing in that style. It's boring—for you and those who have to look at you. If you see yourself as casual-sporty, that doesn't mean you should wear pants and boots every day for every occasion. Casual-sporty does not mean clinging to just one or two expressions of the look. It can mean casual dresses and suits, as well.

It has always seemed to me that dressing in style is more a matter of wearing your *self* than wearing what the fashion press dictates. Finding your individual style-self means having a clear idea of who you are in terms of your *essential* personhood, and realizing that that person changes only in small degrees throughout her whole life. Certainly your age changes, your financial circumstances can change, and even your body will change, but the essential *you* that cries out to be communicated through your clothing really doesn't change through the years. A person who has a "uniform" mentality will wear her prep school and camp uniforms in childhood exactly reflecting her peers' clothing, and then when she grows older, she'll wear, almost exclusively, the little G's, C's, or D's uniform that signifies she's a dues-paying member of the Gucci, Cardin, or Dior group. Blatantly wearing someone else's initials makes a group statement; it says, "I'm the same as everyone else in this group." It says nothing about who you are inside, your own eclectic individuality.

Just as bad is wearing something that's different for the sake of being different. That's a uniform of a different cut. It also says you're unaware of what you are, and are dressing just to be different from everyone else, no matter if it's right for you or not. It just looks bizarre most of the time.

On the other hand there are the truly chic, the truly stylish, who know their own personalities and have translated them into clothing. If you are genuinely versatile, if you see the world in an original way, you'll pick up the options available in the stores and wear them creatively. You can combine fabrics in a surprising and unexpected manner—a velvet blazer with jeans, a beaded evening sweater with wonderfully tailored linen pants. You can make a "suit" from a white lace antique jacket you've picked up in a thrift shop and a navy silk skirt you've resurrected from a two-piece dress bought ten years ago. The possibilities are endless.

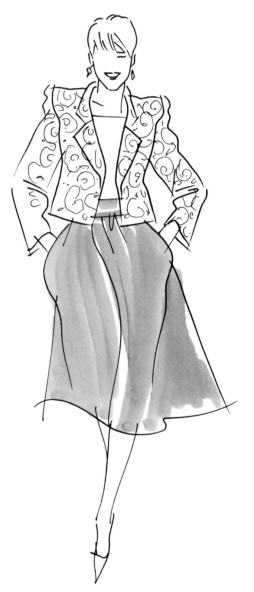

A white lace antique jacket and navy skirt

If you are a woman whose personality cries out for easy, body-conscious clothes that move—because *you* move athletically, professionally, and emotionally—you're going to feel and look stilted and unnatural in starched organdies, perishable velvets, and trendy metallics. For you are the easygoing and comfortable mohair and angora sweaters at night, and the soft and wearable hand-knits, wools, and natural cotton fabrics by day. That doesn't mean you have to eschew designer clothes; it only means that you should choose them when they suit you. The Norma Kamali sweatshirt dresses would look great, for instance, on the fast-moving and easy-living woman and be somehow very out of place on her delicate, fragile, and old-world type sister. Jane Fonda, for instance, looks best when she dresses in a sporty, free-thinking, freshly upbeat way: The image she tried to project many years ago of darkly sensuous glamour was simply silly. Her *self* is leggy, unique, honest, daring; *not* for her the ruffled, extravagantly feminine, the décolleté, the beaded tunics. Instead, intelligent, never gimicky dressing—the sensational silks, the leathers, the casual classics that show off her great body and dramatic appeal. Are you getting the picture? Test yourself. Which would look best on Jane Fonda as she dresses for the Academy Awards:

- a sheer, peachy lace blouse, ruffled organza skirt, and glittery drop earrings

or

- a black tank top studded with unexpected black sequins worn with a long, straight silk skirt?

The latter is more her style, of course; ruffles on Fonda are overkill. On the other hand, a sleek tank top with the unexpected sequins are much more her "dress-up" *self*-expression.

Remember when Nancy Reagan wore knickers to a party in Paris? They may have been fashionable, but they looked absurd because her personal style is simple, classic femininity—and *not* cutesy knickers (more appropriate on a nineteen-year-old horsewoman). You are your own worst fashion enemy when you don't understand your soul . . . when you don't dress in a way that says, "Yes— this is me—really *me*." You can't look self-confident, no matter how much money you spend on clothes, if you dress like a peasant milkmaid when the essential *you* cries out with unmistakable clarity, "I am a big-city sophisticate!"

Being stylish in clothes doesn't mean imitating, but I really do believe that you can learn what's terrific for you by being observant. You have to be aware of what kinds of fabrics, colors, and cuts flatter your particular coloring and body structure—as well as your life style and personality. You have to learn what's *available*. And even though this statement may seem to contradict what I've said earlier, you really have to be knowledgeable about fashion *trends*. That does not mean you have to slavishly follow the dictates of the designers; it just means that very short skirts look crude if the general look is sleek, longer hems. That means that puffy shoulders look pretentious if a natural shoulder line is the last word in *Vogue*.

So, what do you do to learn how to choose clothing with style? Invest in the fashion magazines to start, because they give you an *idea* of what's available and what's new. However, doing everything the designers and the fashion arbiters suggest will make you anonymous. It's like signing a petition—you get lost in the signatures. *But*, if you're able to read selectively, you choose what's terrific for you, discarding the styles that don't give the message you wish to send out. You can discover combinations that are perfect for you if you watch carefully: You may be a red-worn-with-purple type, but you may not know it unless you see it on a model in *Vogue* or *Harper's Bazaar*. You may never have even thought of wearing red with purple, but suddenly you see a woman who reminds you of you jumping out of an advertisement, you *recognize* her as having a quality that's peculiarly yours, and, *voilà*—red and purple together becomes a look uniquely yours even though your mother told you never, never to wear red and purple together because they clash . . . and until this day you never have.

Another way to develop a sense of individual style is to keep an eye on people you think always look wonderful. I am not saying *copy* someone else's personal style—just observe it, adopt what's good for you, discard what's not. That's the "Having a Mentor" type of education, and if it works in careers and in the arts, why shouldn't it be meaningful in dress as well? Everyone needs role models, whether they are mothers, favorite writers, politicians, or best friends. That's how you learn—when you select people to admire and base your goals on. Imitation is blind; style is accomplished with careful observation. For instance, I am in the world of high-fashion modeling, but high fashion does not necessarily mean style. I am paid by manufacturers to wear their clothing—whether or not I personally like their choices for me. But that's business. When it comes to choosing my own wardrobe, it's not business—it's my life. Although fashion is my career, I had to carefully develop a personal *style* sense that was innately *Cristina*. As much of a paradox as it sounds, I looked around at others to do that. One woman I greatly admired for her sense of high style and flair was Joanna Carson. She seemed to choose the fabrics and cuts of clothing that were most like my life and personality. So I watched her carefully, saw how she blended various colors and textures . . . and I put myself in her boots when I went shopping. I would say to myself, "Would Joanna wear this?" When the answer seemed an unequivocal *yes*, I considered the style for myself. Much of the time I found I was able to express my own self very well in these cuts and fabrics that looked well on her. Then I had to get more selective. For instance, I found that Joanna looked elegant in bold prints, in yellows and oranges. When I chose a dress in a strong orange print, the dress wore me. It simply didn't work. So I had to look for dresses that were basically solid colors rather than prints—and in reds and blacks rather than oranges and yellows. Even though the cuts and fabrics of Joanna's clothes were right for me, some of the colors were not. Also she can wear feathers and ribbons and scallops on the hems of ball gowns, but I can't; I am more *Cristina* in straight and simple clothes. Beading beats scallops on gowns for me. And, thus, I educated myself. By checking out the choices of women whose clothes sense I admired, I learned to modify and choose what was fine on me. By reading fashion magazines, by watching others, my own style began to emerge as clearly as though it were given to me as a present when I was born. Today, I can look at

Olivia Newton-John, admire her softly pastel angora sweaters and her headbands and still know instantly that although angora and headbands are very Newton-John, they are very nutty on Ferrare.

Train your eye by observing the rich at play. I know that money doesn't buy taste or style, but often money can buy the services of the professionals who do have taste and whose style may be an expression of your instincts. Have a drink in a restaurant where you can't afford to eat; walk on an elegant avenue in your city and watch how the monied people express their taste and judge what you think appropriate to copy—and what you think tacky beyond all measure. It takes time, observation, and practice for your own fashion voice to emerge.

A very basic element of that voice is consistency. That doesn't mean you have to dress sporty all the time or formally all the time. It means that people should know what to expect of you because your taste is reliably constant whether you're shopping for clothing or furniture. People would be very surprised if they saw me in a blouse with glittering spangles sewn on—just as they'd be surprised if they came to my home and saw metallic glitters woven into the kitchen flooring. It's not *consistent* with the style I've chosen for myself. What would be appropriate for me, what people would expect to see me wear in a blouse would be simple, a tailored natural fabric; on a kitchen floor, they'd expect to see hand-painted tiles rather than glittering linoleum. It's not that tiles are necessarily better than linoleum—it's just that my personal style *reads* tiles-not-linoleum in my kitchen. It's *my* look.

Nevertheless, having said all this, I don't think it's contradictory to say that there are some style basics about shopping and dressing that are consistently true for many elegant women. I've been in the fashion business for a long time, and I seem to have picked up a fairly good sense of how to dress with a reasonable amount of common sense "smarts" and good taste. Let me tell you some of the things I've learned as an educated consumer and as a fashion model that might act as background to your own development of personal dressing style. To begin with, one has to *get to* the clothes.

Where to Shop

I didn't always make a whole lot of money and I had to be quite careful about spending too much on clothing. It was a dilemma because I'd learned at an early age to buy *good*. Cheap fabrics and hastily thrown together designs simply didn't hack it for me. And so I learned how to buy *good*, cheaply. The rules of thumb for buying good, cheaply are to:

SHOP THE SALES. You get a far better buy going into a very fine store on Fifth Avenue (or Main Street or the Champs Élysées or wherever you happen to live) when they're having their twice-a-year sales than going into a tacky store where the merchandise is cheap but poorly made and not design conscious. The best time to find the yearly sales are after Christmas and in August. When I buy shoes, for instance, I almost always go to a fine store like Charles Jourdan where I can pick up a two-hundred-dollar pair of shoes for eighty dollars at sale time. They'll last forever and look wonderful in contrast to the cheap shoes I might buy for thirty dollars, which will last for a season (maybe) and always look just short of great. Clothes in the finest department stores are reduced sometimes up to 50 and 60 percent, so a hundred-dollar silk blouse ends up being fifty dollars, and its color is more true and its styling more detailed than the thirty-dollar blouse in a cheaper-priced store.

SHOP THE DISCOUNT HOUSES. In every community there's a store called Remin's or Loehmann's or Bolton's or Insomnia, where designer and other high-priced clothing is sold at great savings. This is because the store buyers purchase in bulk, or last season's merchandise, or clothing that has *imperceptible* faults (a button that fell off and can easily be resewn, a hem that's hanging slightly). Whatever the reason, the store has been able to get its merchandise cheaper, and you're the winner if you pick up an original Cardin $350 suit for $100. You may have to put up with communal dressing rooms and far less personalized sales help, but if you have an eye for style, you can buy a whole season's wardrobe at a fraction of the price you'd pay for it in the elegant stores. Often discount stores have no-return or limited return policies, so your option to change your mind about your purchase is narrowed; still, the huge savings are clearly worth it. The materials, the cuts, the styles will be infinitely superior to those found in the cheap stores.

TIP: Find out when the discount store in your neighborhood gets its shipments; being there the day the new clothes arrive gives you a far greater choice.

SHOP THE AUCTION HOUSES. Ask the better auction houses in your neighborhood when they next plan an "old clothes" sale. I have found fabulous hand-beaded gowns that must have originally cost five thousand dollars for two or three hundred dollars. I've bought the most magnificent lace for fifty dollars that had to cost five hundred dollars new, and when I added it to an old black wool dress, I had an outfit that would have been outrageously expensive to purchase. Auction houses don't have such creative instincts, but if you do, you can buy, for example, for thirty dollars, a size ten, white, lacy organdy nightgown that a short lady in 1890 went to sleep in. For another fifty dollars, you can bring the nightgown to a dressmaker who will alter it to fit size eight (you), and for a grand total of eighty dollars, you have the most exquisite summer party dress that would cost close to six hundred dollars in a fashionable store. In auction sales, I have bought magnificent braided velvet jackets, fur coats, beaded bags, embroidered blouses, satin ball gowns. What's more, in auction houses you can buy original and classic dresses by Balenciaga, Fortuny, Chanel (so unique and so well made they'd be impossible to criticize) for a fraction of their original cost. Last year, I wore a black beaded dress from the thirties to a charity ball. My dress was unusual—I knew it! I felt unique.

A stunning party dress from an antique lace nightgown

SHOP THE DEPARTMENT STORES. FIND THE READY-TO-WEAR DEPARTMENTS OF THE COUTURE DESIGNERS. Halston, Sonia Rykiel, Albert Nipon, John Anthony, Anne Klein, and other high-priced designers have just started to knock off their own fabulous (and fabulously expensive) designs at ready-made prices. Instead of paying $2,500 for a suit, you can now own a designer suit for, say, under $125. You're getting the same impeccable taste and design of the famous designers with perhaps a *little* less lush fabric. It's the way to go—buying an extraordinarily lower-priced version of extraordinary clothing.

SHOP THE VINTAGE CLOTHING STORES. Each age had its own palette of colors, textures, and styles and the true woman of style in the eighties knows that the forties and fifties and twenties and thirties were timeless. Looks keep coming full circle, and you can mix and match the old with the new for true eclecticism. A forties beaded cashmere sweater can look marvelous with silk pants. A thirties man's satin cummerbund can dress up an eighties wool shift. Even women who have a surplus of money to spend on their clothing often haunt the vintage clothing stores. Endless unique variations are yours for the putting together.

SHOP THE DRESSMAKERS. When I was little, my mother made all my clothes. They cost less than any of my friends' clothes, but I was always the best dressed, and now I *know* why. My clothes fit me. They were designed with *me* in mind. I've always remembered that, so today I keep a dressmaker's dummy of me in the basement. Actually, I keep two dummies—a thin one and a heavier

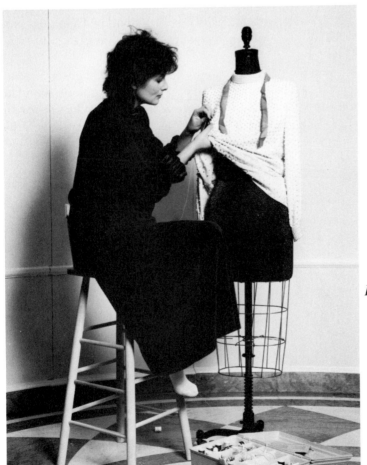

A forties beaded sweater with silk pants for the eighties

Fastening loose beads on an antique tunic

one. I use one or the other depending on the state of my diet. In every town there is always a local dressmaker (who will probably charge less than it would cost you to buy a good dress) to *make* a dress designed for you and fit *on* you. Often such a dressmaker can create a dress you love from a picture you bring him or her. You don't need your own dressmaking dummy if you have someone else do the work, but I find that I save a lot on tailoring bills by putting a new dress that needs a hem right on the dummy and hemming it myself. That way I always have the length exactly correct.

SHOP THE SHOWROOMS. Here's a little-known tip. The major fashion designers sometimes have days when they open their showrooms to the public (as a goodwill gesture or perhaps to sell slightly model-worn merchandise). You might not get a discount on such clothing, but you will save the considerable department store markup. Now every designer does not do this; however, if you have a favorite one and a special occasion coming up, try calling the offices of the designer in your nearest large city (you won't find Bill Blass or Yves Saint Laurent offices in Lewisburg, Pennsylvania) and just ask if the public is ever permitted to browse. Naturally each designer has fashion shows to which the press, the store buyers, and a select audience of friends are invited—but that's not what I'm talking about. Even if you could wangle an invitation to such a show, it's not the time to try on merchandise.

If you're determined to have a designer dress that you can't afford with a store markup, and you've been told that there are no "open to the public" days, your only other alternative is to scout around for someone to arrange a private visit for you. Do you have a pal who is
- a high-fashion model,
- a press person in the area of fashion or life styles,
- a department store buyer,
- a steady customer of the designer?

Perhaps she/he can arrange an entry to the showroom for you. It's worth a try.

So buy *good*, even if you have to buy less; even if you have to go farther for those good things. You just can't look stylish in clothes made with shiny, tawdry fabrics that are shoddily put together. Your clothing gives off a message of style, of class, that's as loud as anything you might write or say about yourself.

When to Shop

It's simple. You shop when you are hungry. Hunger does wonders to keep you alert and sharp. Your stomach looks flatter, your whole body feels less bloated and your clothes fit better. Shopping for clothing is precisely the opposite of shopping for food, which you do when you're full: Happily sated bellies are terrific in getting you to pass the Hershey's chocolate bar department. Somehow shopping for clothes with an empty stomach changes your whole attitude.

With Whom to Shop

NO ONE. Always shop alone. Other people distract you, make you feel guilty for keeping them waiting. What's more, you'll find yourself developing better style judgment if you don't have your aunt, mother, and best friend offering opinions on everything you try. Even shopping with the woman you've chosen as a fashion mentor can be a mistake because you'll tend to follow her directives—instead of developing your own taste, using her taste just as a focal point. Shopping alone means just you in the dressing room—and not a salesperson, either. Never trust anyone who says, "Oh, darling, it's simply fabulous on you." Salespeople often work on commission, and they're interested in the number of sales they make—not your good looks. Most always they lie through their teeth. If you don't believe me, try on something in shiny chartreuse with ill fit and bad design. "Oh, darling, it's fabulous" will no doubt be the refrain. If you have to think about something a lot, it's probably not for you. Ninety percent of the time, you'll get it home and hate it—or not love it, at best. But if you put it on and it's absolutely to die from right away—even if it's a little small, it's probably super for you. What's more, it'll give you an incentive to diet.

How to Use the System

The biggest error women make is to shop in only those stores they can realistically afford. You should *buy* your clothes in the stores within your budget, but you should not *shop* in those places. You can learn how to best judge good fabric, cut, design, and color by shopping at the stores that provide quality merchandise because their customers can afford it and demand it. We have a wonderful system in America—we can try on million-dollar outfits and ideas for free. We can put thousands of dollars of clothing and accessories on our backs and walk out without spending a dime (assuming we've taken the clothes off first). And what have we gained? Plenty. The ability to distinguish between shoddy and chic. Classic and trendy. Workmanship and slapdash. And even though you can also buy outrageously kitschy clothing in a posh, expensive store, the only way to learn what looks good, what works, and what options are available is to experiment, and the way to do that is to play in a large department store. Naturally one has to play cricket and not take up too much of any salesperson's time. It also is civilized not to wear a whole lot of makeup that can come off on the clothes you're trying on. What you do is this: On a day when your hair looks good (don't try on clothes when your hair looks crummy because the rest of you often follows suit) and you feel slender and pretty, go to the designer department of a large store and try on clothes you *know* you'd never in a million years buy because they're too expensive. Put together outfits that are pure fancy. Experiment with scarves, belts, different hair looks. If you've always thought you'd look dreadful in knits and for that reason have never had one, try on knits galore. Analyze. Look at every angle. Look at yourself with a critical eye. Pick outfits you'd never pick if you were actually buying.

Are you wasting time? Absolutely not. What you're doing is courting fashion to develop style. If you only try on when you intend to buy, you tend to limit your horizons to what you can afford and not to what looks great. But if you give yourself the present of a free hand every once in a while, you look at yourself and your *possibilities* differently. Afterward you can translate what you like and what you can't afford to what you like and can afford. Once you know that knits are a viable option, having tried on a very good one, you may gravitate toward a knit when you're out to make a real purchase. We all tend to buy the same thing, over and over. If you *love* black turtlenecks, I guarantee that you have too many of them in your closet. In terms of colors and styles, most of us look for that one dynamite outfit that did so much for us when we were eighteen—and we keep looking for it when we're thirty and forty and fifty—*and we keep buying it*, in one form or another. Experimenting gets us out of that bind, opens the door to change. Style in dressing, you see, has to do with vital, unmistakable assurance—as well as the clothes. When you buy an outfit, you ought to think, "Now, how many ways can I wear this?" When you are in the habit of selecting with an assured confidence, you allow yourself to make changes. And small changes lead to bigger changes—and before you know it, you're the person with the most interesting look in the room. You can wear a beaded tunic over black silk pants and look more stylish than the woman with the most elaborate gown—but first you have to know that fabulous beaded tunics exist somewhere: You learn it by checking out department stores—when you're *not* buying.

Become Important to the Salesperson

Salespeople can really help to make your life easier when shopping. There's a knack to getting them to adopt your problems as their problems. First of all, you have to get their attention. Most of the time, it's as simple as talking to them as if they're people and you *care*—no one ever does. "Good morning, how *are* you today?" Smile, maybe even touch, then ask your question. Never let a salesperson snub you, especially if she's not busy; personalize your query before you express your needs. Your purpose is to get the salesperson to work *for* you, and graciousness means attention to the fact that the salesperson is human, not a robot. Salespeople should be able to
- give you directions regarding where to find merchandise;
- make suggestions as to size;
- tell you the specific characteristics of the merchandise (is it washable, durable, and so on).

A salesperson's *opinion* on *how* something looks on you should never be sought because that opinion is not really meaningful; she may be pushing a sale because of a hoped-for commission, uninterested in your good looks, unqualified to know what's stylish and what isn't, and generally not to be trusted . . . even if she means well.

Playing in department stores every once in a while, and utilizing the merchandise and the sales help properly, is a style-expanding thing to do. It helps you to dress rich and dress classy, even if you don't have a healthy stock portfolio.

On Trend Setting

Style can mean originality of thought also, and that can result in setting trends. But trend setting doesn't imply kooky clothing. Your clothes can be nonconformist and distinctive without being bizarre. Liza Minnelli, for instance, set a "tuxedo" trend. She's always enjoyed wearing man-tailored clothes, and that suits her style of life besides. As a dancer, she can't get too locked into clothes that don't move easily, and men's clothing doesn't bind. It seemed as if everyone was sporting tuxedos after *Cabaret* hit the movie theaters. Isabella Rossellini, a top fashion model, seems cut out to wear clothing from another time, another era. Her very nature calls for gentle, aristocratic-looking clothing, and if a trend for the old-fashioned look appears in the next few months, Isabella's unique way of modeling gaslight-era fashion will probably have a lot to do with it.

Being a trend setter has to do with wearing your own look with energy and confidence . . . even if that look is not on the fashion pages of *Harper's Bazaar*. Forcing a unique look just for the sake of being different doesn't cut it when you're talking true style.

Dressing Easy

In today's modern world, most of us like to dress down, dress easy. Dressing easy doesn't mean dressing sloppy. For instance, I love warm-up suits, even if I'm not warming up for anything in particular. Who says you have to be the tennis champ in order to wear her clothes? Warm-up suits come in luxuriant colors, they always look neat, and they're snugly warm in the winter. Jeans are not necessarily the most comfortable item in the world, even though we've been brainwashed to believe that. And jeans do tend to look seedy, sloppy. For an easy movie or a lunch date with my friends, I love a basic pair of pants, tailored impeccably. Add a pretty silk blouse, a smashing belt, top the whole thing off with some interesting earrings and you're ready to go anywhere. Scarves are not big in my wardrobe; I find them cumbersome. If you don't have a real knack of tying a scarf with just that right dash of *éclat* the scarf detracts from your style rather than adds to it. Materials that go with dressing easy are jersey, cotton, and cotton duck in the summertime, light, swingy wools, gabardines, and corduroys in the fall, and heavier wools, velvets, and knits in the colder weather.

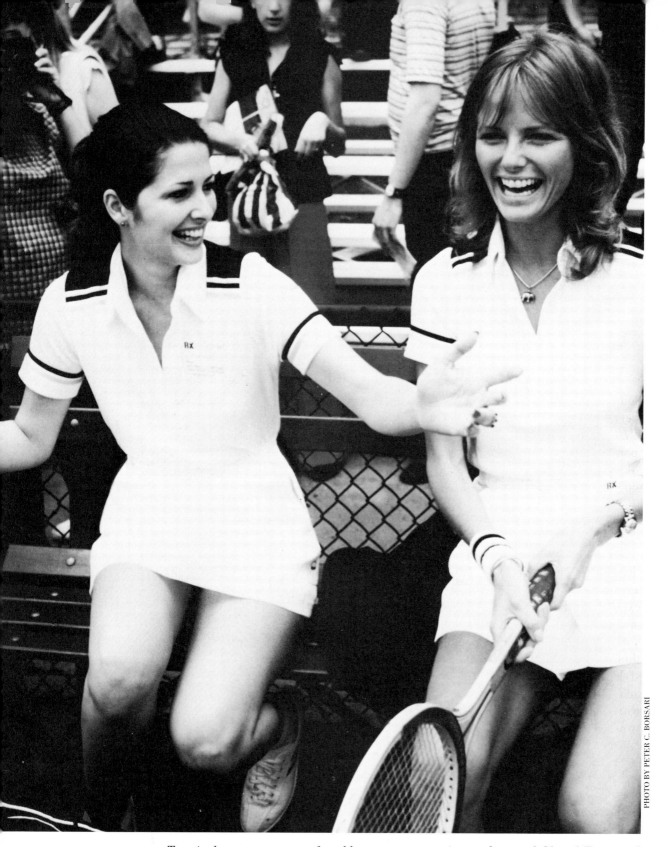

Tennis dresses are as comfortable as warm-up suits, and my pal Cheryl Tiegs and I wear them for tennis and for "hanging out."

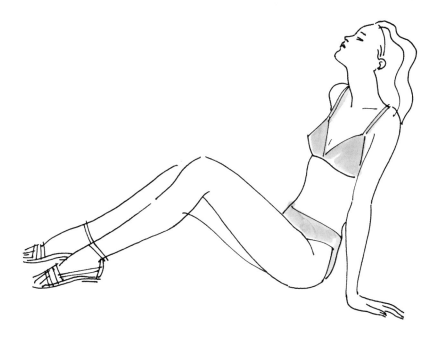

To me, dressing easy with style means dressing appropriately—using common sense. For instance, on the beach I'd never in a million years wear high heels with a bathing suit unless I wanted to look like something out of *The Dukes of Hazzard*. Shoes for the beach must be flat—the sand, the situation, *insists* upon it. But you can buy a strappy, sexy-looking sandal (straps tied around your ankles are always sexy looking), and if your feet are appealingly manicured, you're looking good!

DOSE OF PIZZAZZ

Whenever I'm dressing easy, I find that adding something with flair to even a conservative outfit gives it interest and excitement. For instance, that same pair of simple black pants can be topped with a narrow snakeskin belt that adds something a plain leather belt couldn't. It's style. A creamy white tailored blouse and a black wool skirt are brought to life with, say, a red-red leather bag—or a two-tone pump.

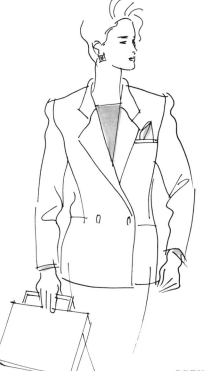

A classic all-day, all-night blazer

MOVE INTO EVENING WITH EASE

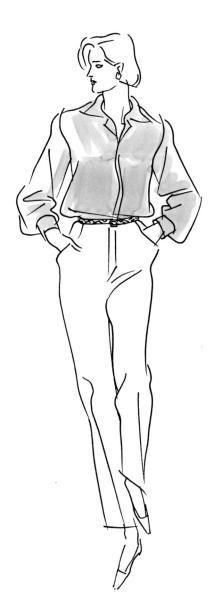

Nighttime elegance can be easy also: Well-tailored pants in crepe or soft wool, a paisley blouse, or a colorful sweater can be smashing. And take jackets or blazers: When you buy a timeless, well-tailored classic, it can see you through your day, through dinner, through theater—through any casual time. Classic jackets are *not* puffy sleeved, or double breasted, or any particular fashion whim of the moment. They're fluid and straight and simple and can be dressed up or down with uncomplicated accessories—a great gold chain, an art deco rhinestone pin on a lapel. Dressing easy with style, I suppose, means having the classics in your closet—with maybe an aberration or so that bows to the current fashion, like a peasant skirt or a puffy-sleeved blouse —for fun and variety's sake.

Dressing Up

GO FOR THE UNEXPECTED

It's a sense of surprise that gives class to clothes. Happy surprise—not nightmare surprise. For instance, if you have a simple black wool/satin tuxedo jacket you've resurrected from a suit you used to love, you can use it as an elegant top to a sexy Charmeuse slip dress; *or*, you can wear the classic jacket with an unusual texture, like a lace skirt, for a very formal look. At an auction I once bought a wonderful black beaded dress that was far too short because it was probably worn by a four-foot woman in 1859. I bought a piece of black fox fur, had a local dressmaker sew it on the hem, and the dress was a one-of-a-kind miracle. Dressing up is truly great fun. What's more, I think that when you dress up, you should expect other people to pay attention to you. What's the point of all those terrific clothes if no one notices? And that's where attitude comes in. Style is a matter of attitude as well as clothing choices. If you *think* you're terrific, hold your head high, and walk with grace, you probably will *look* terrific. My daughter, Kathryn, learned this at an early age, and I love to see that certain sense of quiet confidence. Once, as she pranced out the door to a fellow four-year-old's birthday party, I was taken by her charm and carriage. "You know, Kathryn," I said to her little gray sweatsuit–dressed self, "You really have quite a bit of style." She looked at me with great seriousness. "Thank you," she said simply. With style.

THE ONE ALWAYS-WORKS OUTFIT

It's the nature of my business to have a lot of clothes in my closet, but I rarely seem to wear the collection I've amassed. Even though I'm photographed in the most fabulous clothes of the year, for myself I keep coming back to the "One Great Outfit" that always works—my favorite pair of black velvet jeans,

Black pants dressed down

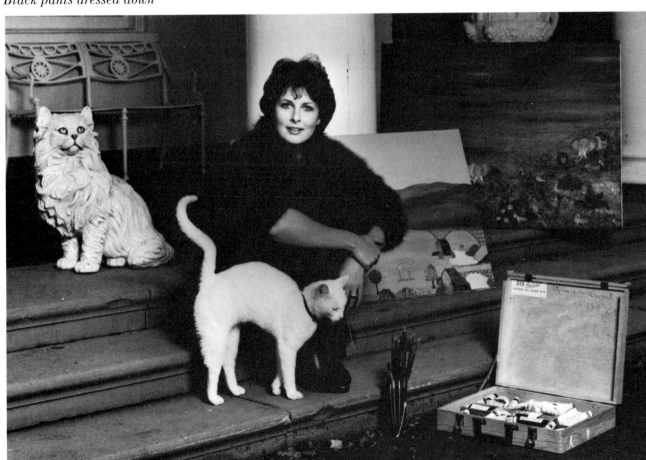

which I dress up or down with silk blouses or casual sweaters, depending on where I'm headed. It's right for a friend's house, for a cocktail party, for dinner. I wear many variations of the outfit in silk pants and a sweater for the evening, and crepe pants and a blouse for shopping. For me, style means what my husband, John, once told me: "Never wear anything that wears you." Perhaps others can get away with kooky wild clothing, but my style decrees simplicity.

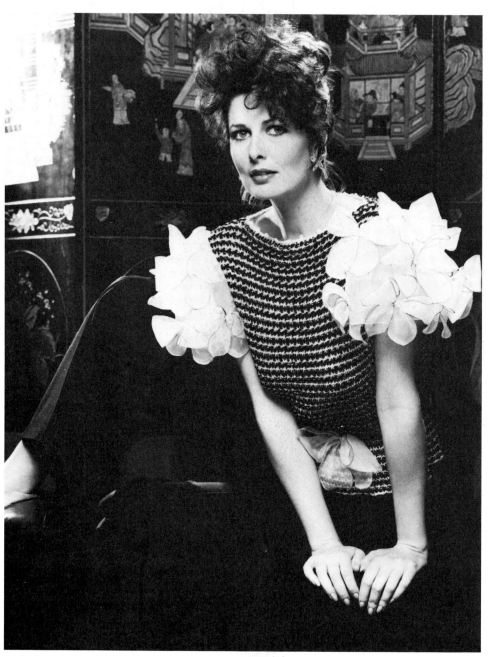

Black pants dressed up

Personal Style

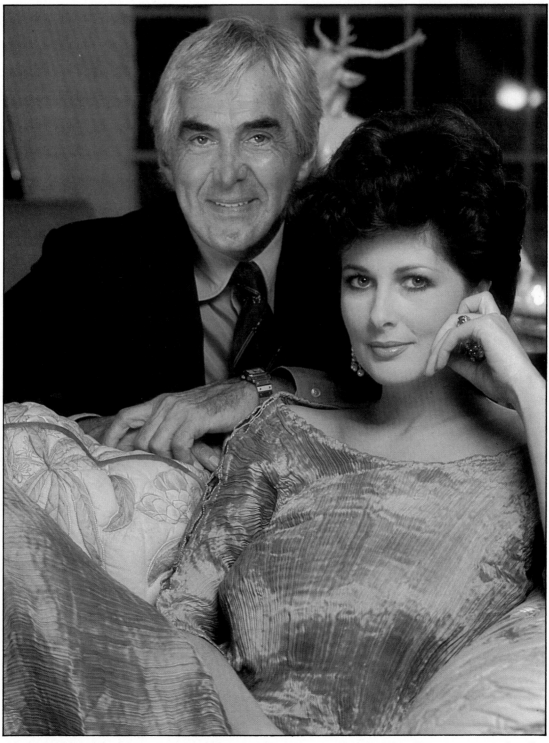

John and I dressed for a party. I'm wearing my priceless antique Fortuny gown that I bought for a less-than-priceless price at auction.

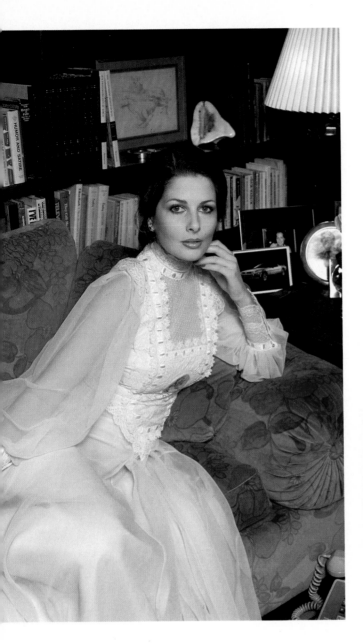

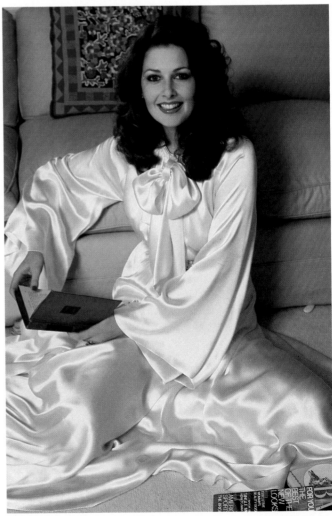

Two options for long hair: swept back and flowing.

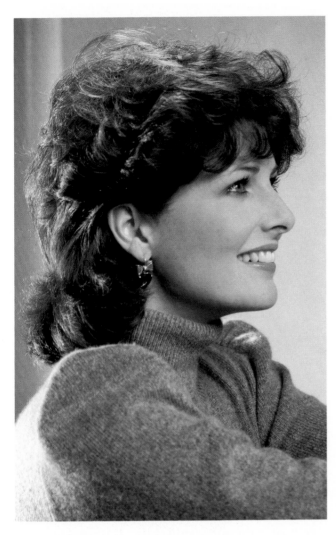

Two options for shorter hair: caught up with a comb behind each ear and fluffed in an aureole of curls.

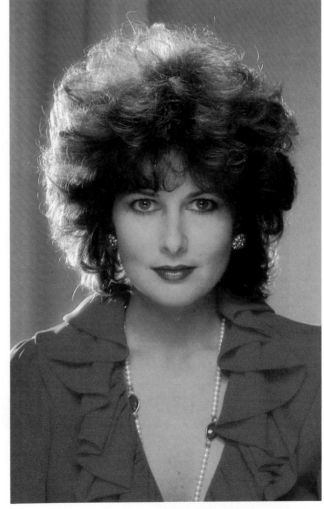

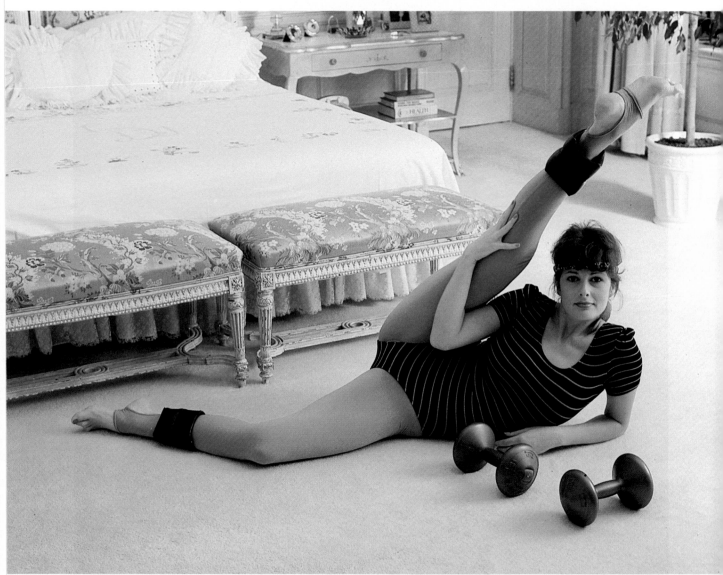

Staying in shape at home.

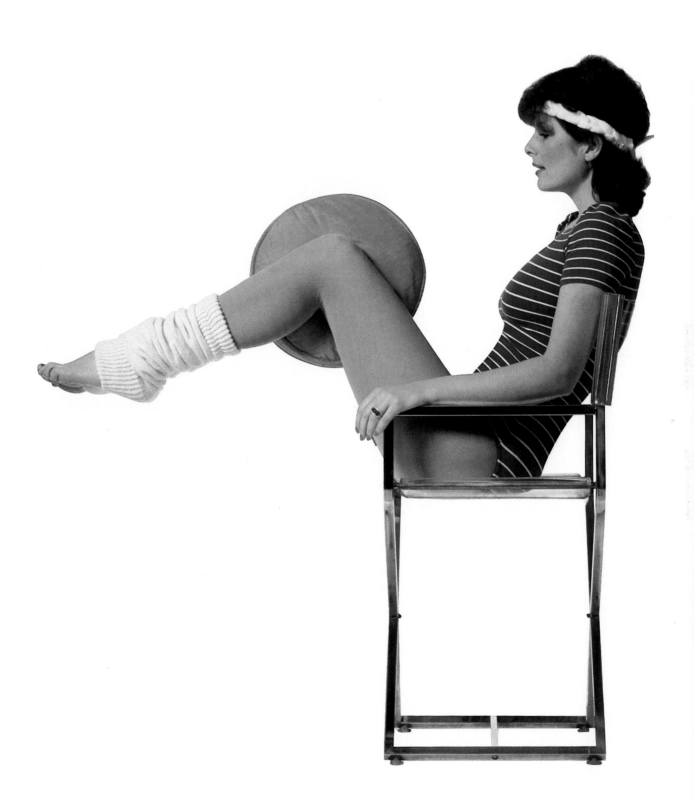

*Artist at work—and visitor.
Did you ever see such a
wonderful cat?*

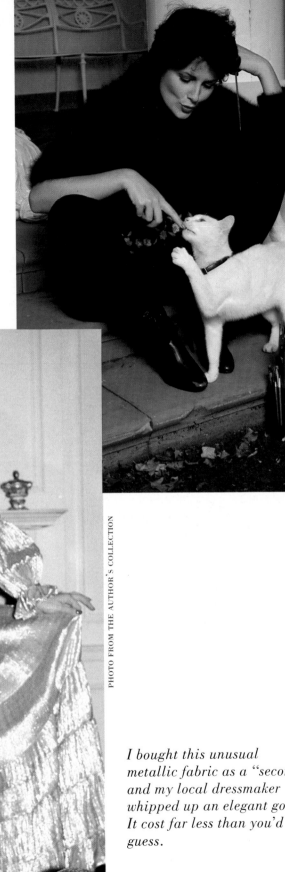

*I bought this unusual
metallic fabric as a "second"
and my local dressmaker
whipped up an elegant gown.
It cost far less than you'd
guess.*

ACCESSORIES: THE EXCEPTION

They don't have to be so simple because they're sparse. I love to wear, for instance, one terrific dangling earring. I love something dramatically unusual like an ornate silver match case from the 1800s worn on a chain around my neck. Accessories shouldn't be layered on (nothing really should, I think—that adds bulk and width more than interest) but chosen carefully and individually for prettiness and excitement. Sometimes an accessory can be a color, and if it's bright and bold enough, you don't need much to create an impact. Red, for instance, is a high-spirited accessory color and a body-skimming white jersey dress with a red sash (if you have the body to go with the skimming) can be a blast of color contrast that is far more dramatic than a fussy floral print, for example. An accessory can be a style freshener; it can add drama to your dress.

Dressing for Success

Practically a catch phrase in our time, dress for success has come to mean dressing conservatively. But, no matter what your job is, dressing for success doesn't mean drab colors and three-piece suits exclusively. When you're playing to win, business suits can have a piece of the unexpected in them too. For instance, the classic navy double-breasted jacket and white blouse look okay but boring with a regular skirt. Add a calf-skimming skirt, a great neck piece, an interesting bag and belt with the same jacket and blouse and you have style—something that works as you work. You can be terribly businesslike with an un-uniform look. Suits of different lengths and dresses with different shapes don't stereotype you. If you select clothes that are uniforms, you become faceless, selfless. The point is to be individual even in stock situations. If you are aiming for a promotion, dressing in the little brown suit with the pearls every day won't necessarily help that advancement along. Neither will dressing in outrageous raspberry culottes. *But*, the little brown suit *with* an outrageous raspberry blouse may just be the ticket to convince the boss (along with your skills) that you're *interesting*. It's the little bland pilot fish that swim alongside the streamlined sharks of chic who get lost in the movements of the tide. The sharks prevail because of their flair—size is secondary. Sometimes the biggest fish in the sea are the clumsiest. Sometimes they're not. It's a matter of style. It works for people also.

Blazer with calf skimming skirt and great neck piece

Nobody's Perfect

Jackie Onassis has skinny bowlegs. And very big feet. Liza Minnelli has a *very* short neck. I have a *very* full rear view. If you take a sharp good look in the mirror at yourself—with and without clothes—you can clearly evaluate your less-than-fabulous figure. Then learn to compensate, camouflage, point to the things that *are* fabulous. By camouflage, I don't mean hide. You really can't hide completely. Men who wear bad toupees are fooling no one. Far better, if you have a balding head, to grow a beard and call attention to another part of the forest. Far better, if you have a bulging stomach, to eschew tight blood- and breath-constricting girdles and, instead, wear waistless A-line dresses, overblouses, and tunics. You cannot a bulging stomach hide with a flouncy dirndl dress. You cannot a short neck hide with an elaborate, chunky choker necklace. Far better to opt for a dipping V-neck, a long, low, simple chain necklace, a low-slung scarf to pull the eye down.

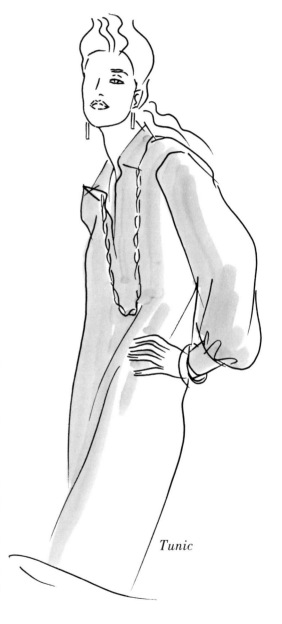

Tunic

What follows are some suggestions on how to create different proportions from the ones with which you were born. Try them, and, above all, don't despair if you were born without a waist. Find your personal style in dressing that makes no-waists something adorable.

YOU'RE A LITTLE CHUNKIER THAN YOU'D LIKE? Avoid bows and puffs and ruffles—anything that sits like a bump on a dress. Avoid tight clothes as much as you avoid tents . . . neither will make you look slimmer. Pleats at the waistbands of skirts and pants are out and so are the dumb turquoise polyester pants with a stretch waistband. See what the fashion designers in the large-size departments are coming out with. Tunics are great—not in mad, floral Omar-the-Tentmaker specials, but in pretty colors, delicate prints. Don't stick to navies and blacks, which don't make you look any thinner, really. The point is to try to look terrific—not necessarily sylphlike (which is impossible if you're being honest). Boots should disappear under your skirt and not cut your calf in half. If you have a very limited budget, buy inexpensive, simple fabrics, but splurge on a dynamite, expensively tailored scarf that will make the outfit. Stay away from ugly, mother-of-the-bride mint greens and foam yellows, and make a statement with fabulous plums, charcoals, tweeds. Cute is out and so is ethnic (Guatemalan gauzes, for instance). Sloppy is absolutely out. So are tight belts, bosom-length beads, open-toed shoes. In are suits, shifts, finely mantailored clothes. In are classic pumps, monochromatic colors, longer lengths, fullness at the front of skirts. Out are dirndl skirts, double-breasted anything, baggy pants. In is good taste, above all.

GREAT TIP: Consider having some of your clothes made by the local dressmaker. You can buy natural and wonderful fabrics and have an expert drape them on your own particular shape, which means custom details that flatter *you*. It may not be cheaper than buying good—but it may not be more expensive, either. Best of all: The clothes will be custom fit on you.

BIG BOSOMS. No to low-cut necklines that expose your breasts. *Yes* to turtlenecks, interesting neck scarves and anything that deflects attention from your bustline. Pinched-in waists and wide belts are anathema to large bosoms. Tiny prints, wide-cut jacket armholes and unconstructed clothes are *yes*. Tight T-shirts and clingy fabrics are *no*. Get a great underwire bra; it's worth the investment to get one fitted to your needs.

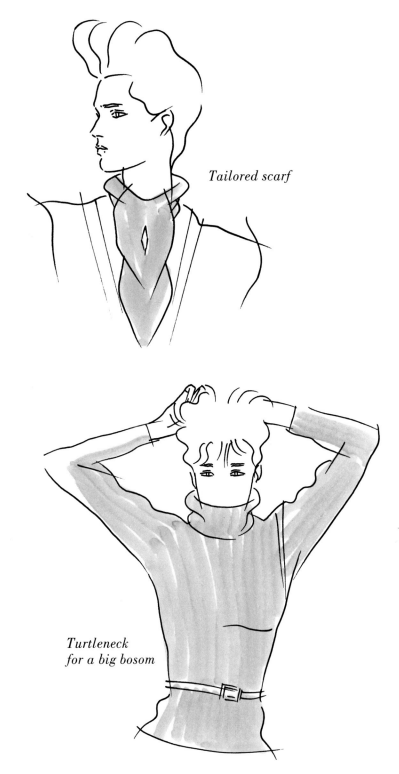

Tailored scarf

Turtleneck for a big bosom

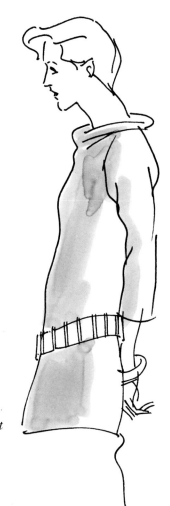

Tunic and hip belt for a short waist

TOO SHORT-WAISTED. Long-drink-of-water lines in clothing are for you. Straight-cut tunics, hip belts, vertical stripes. If you're tall, hip-hugging pants are great; 1920s flapper stuff's for you, also. Don't tuck your shirt into skirts or pants. Contrasting tops and bottoms that point to your waist are to be avoided. Ditto short-cropped jackets and cinched waists. Singles are better than separates; a thin belt, worn below the waist, elongates it. Narrow waistbands rather than wide are better.

LEGS YOU DON'T LOVE. If they're too fat, don't wear white pantyhose. Boots should disappear under your skirt. Soft culottes cut at the calf are great, but *not* if you have very thick ankles. Don't wear your skirts too long, and wear them flared slightly at the hem if your ankles are nonexistent. Pegged pants make heavy legs look like piano legs—stick to straight-leg cuts. Women with very thin legs shouldn't wear dramatic shoes, which give them a spindly, Olive Oyl look— especially if the shoes are of the clunky variety.

YOU'RE VERY TALL

• You carry clothes wonderfully, so be grateful for that. You *can* balance your height with clingy fabrics (only if you're thin) to emphasize curves. Soft, full fabrics also bring out curviness.

• Break the long line with a wide belt or contrasting colors at your waist —one color from head to toe will make you look taller.

• High waistbands on pants and skirts look fine; buttons and bows on tall, reedy women look dopey.

• Hemlines should be longer rather than shorter.

SHOULDERS THAT NEED REDEFINING. Wide shoulders should stay away from padded, ruffled, or cap sleeves. Sleeveless blouses and dresses and dolman sleeves are great. Narrow shoulders should avoid halter tops and dolman droops and concentrate on set-in sleeves and stark, wide collars.

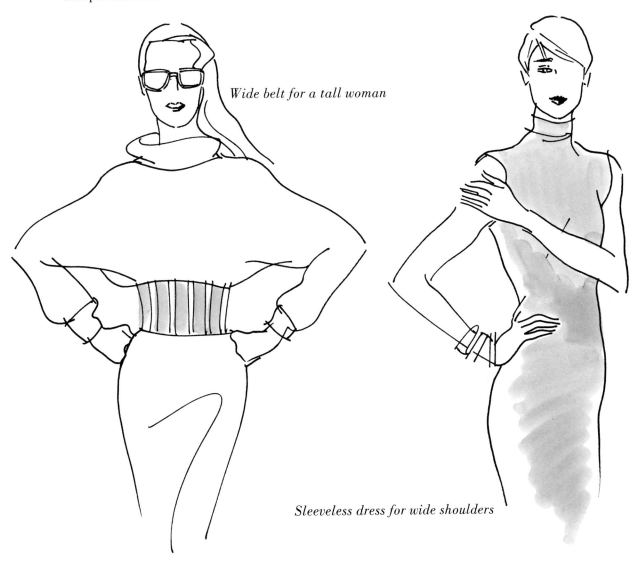

Wide belt for a tall woman

Sleeveless dress for wide shoulders

REAR ADMIRALS. Wide bottoms, bulgy hips (my problem when I overdose on the M & M's) must avoid clingy, silky fabrics. Skirts that are slightly flared and flat pleats (never stitched down) camouflage the bulges. Plaids, tartans, and tight skirts or pants yell that the rear is rearing. Crisp and *good* fabrics (linen, gabardine, heavy cottons that provide body) are best. Anything that gives you an hourglass figure is the pits.

ARM YOURSELF. Heavy or flabby upper arms are nicely hidden in raglan sleeves; loose but not butterfly or kimono sleeves are your optimum choice. Thin arms take on substance with puffier sleeves, gauzier, softer fabrics.

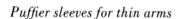
Puffier sleeves for thin arms

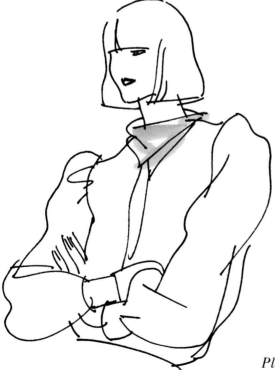

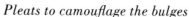
Pleats to camouflage the bulges

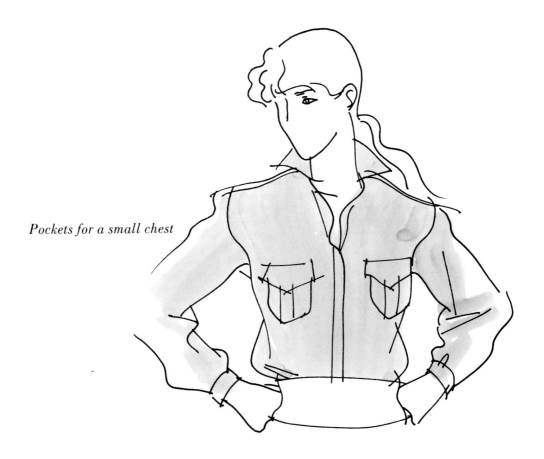

Pockets for a small chest

PANCAKE CHESTS. The good news is that clothes look better, somehow, on women who don't have large bosoms. The bad news is that you don't care—you still wish you were more voluptuous. Try blouses with breast pockets, suit jackets also. Vests are a good look for you. So are diaphanous, transparent organdies and blousier materials. Stay away from clingy jerseys, high-high Peter Pan collars.

FLAT FEET. Whatever you do, don't wear uncomfortable, high-heeled shoes —no matter what the fashion of the day decrees. If your feet hurt and you're thrown off balance, it will show in your face and your attitude. Don't allow designer style to victimize your own central style. Say boots are in—sure, wear boots, but adapt them to a chic, low-heeled version. In the same way that you'd devise a casual sweater and skirt "suit" if sweaters and skirts were in style but tailored suits were your best look, you can modify any shoe trend to *your* heel size.

CANAL-BOAT FEET. If you wear heels, they're more "shortening" than flats. Rounded toes are better than pointies. Wide, horizontally banded sandals in the summer cut length also. So do wedge heels.

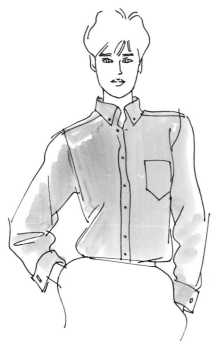

Man-tailored shirt to improve posture

HUNCHBACK OF NOTRE DAME? Bad posture is aging and deforming for thick, thin, short, or tall. Big busts look saggy, no-busts look concave. Tall women look hunched, short women look dumpy—bad posture is a downer for everyone. Exercise and be conscious of your shoulder straightness! Padded shoulders help a little; straight-hanging clothes do also. Scooped and rounded necks are bad; man-tailored shirts are better; tunics are very good.

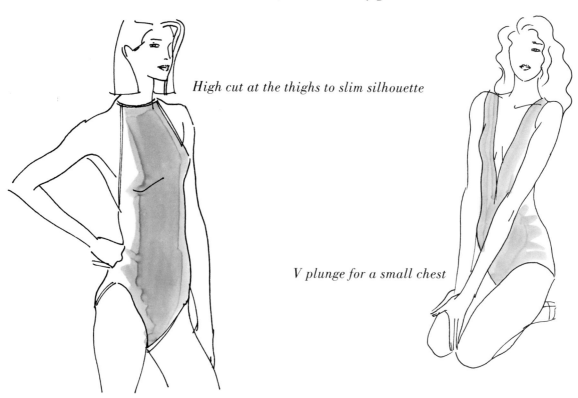

High cut at the thighs to slim silhouette

V plunge for a small chest

NOBODY'S PERFECT AT THE BEACH, FOR SURE. It's the one place where it's really hard to camouflage imperfection. Still, there are some things you can do to help, and when you shop for a bathing suit, keep these points in mind.

Big, Sturdy, Hefty Legs. A high cut at the thighs slims the silhouette. A high cut at the neck gives a longer, leaner look to legs, also. A one-piece suit is a must—stay away from bikinis.

Flat Chests or Broad Shoulders. Try a halter maillot—cut down to *there* in a V plunge. You can definitely carry it.

Small Chest, Small Hips, Small Waist. Only you can wear a bikini

Big Bust. An underwire halter top minimizes the bust. To call attention to the rest of the body, a one-piece suit in one rich, dark color is best. Avoid florals and any big print.

Small Top, Broad Bottom (your classic pear). Try a classic tank with, again, those high-cut legs.

The Really Big Woman. Don't give up your beach fun and, whatever you do, don't try to hide in a large, shapeless, navy-blue skirted tent. Instead of disappearing on the scene, you'll look like a large, navy-blue rock, blaringly large and styleless on the pale beach. If you wear a bathing suit with a flounced skirt, it

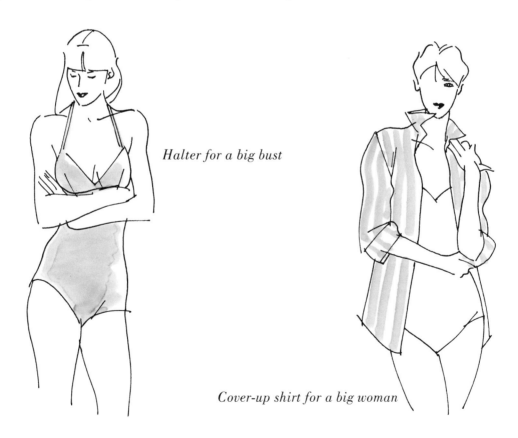

Halter for a big bust

Cover-up shirt for a big woman

won't hide you or make you look thinner. Better still, wear a smart, simple one-piece suit with a stunning cover-up shirt. If you dress like your grandmother, you won't necessarily look any slimmer. Chic is in—in *every* size.

TIP: Stay away from cotton, which tends to sag and get waterlogged when wet. Better (for every size) are the synthetic fabrics in bathing suits.

Remember, style emanates from the head and from the attitude, and although a bathing suit is not your happiest clothing choice, your confidence and humor count more than your girth.

OVER FIFTY? Even if you weigh the same as you did at twenty, your body has changed, your face has changed, and the way you dress should also change. There's no question that you can still be gorgeous—maybe even more gorgeous than ever before, but let's face it, a different kind of gorgeous. It's just not seemly to wear see-through blouses, skintight jeans and skirts that are mini even if mini is in. Flimsy, delicate fabrics that cling to the body are just gauche and do little for middle-age midriff. Bikinis on the beach don't look terrific, unless you *really* do defy the years and have your adolescent firmness as well as thinness intact. V-necks on dresses and blouses are flattering—they elongate the neck and give a graceful look to the whole torso. Take a look at women of high style who are over fifty: Dina Merrill, Katharine Hepburn, Diana Vreeland, Eileen Ford. You wouldn't catch them dead in a tacky clinging fabric, a too-revealing neckline. They're quietly chic in tunics, low-waisted dresses, oversize sweaters. Not a teeny bow anywhere. No gingham.

Style Away from Home

In the good old days travel usually meant unwinding on an ocean liner with clothes hanging neatly in closets until arrival. In the real world of today, travel often means many hours in a plane, bus or car with your clothes bunched in suitcases. Over the years, I've developed packing smarts and I'd like to share them with you.

Pack Smart

The travel books tell you to pack polyester. Yecch! Polyester says *tourist* . . . tasteless, and hot—all the tags you don't need yourself labeled with. Polyester doesn't wrinkle, but it strangles. You could swelter in Rome wearing polyester. Instead, pack cotton, knits, wool jerseys, natural fabrics that *breathe*—in the winter or the summer.

   • So your garments won't crease, place plastic or tissue paper over and in between *everything.*

• Don't schlep heavy winter coats. Instead, a chic raincoat will do for dress-up or rain wear. A zip-in lining or inventive layering underneath will keep out the cold.

• Plastic, zippered bags are great for organizing—especially when you have to dash from hotel to hotel and don't have the time or inclination to pack and unpack everything. One for underwear, one for cosmetics, one for medications, one for blouses, sweaters—you get the idea—then almost everything is compartmentalized and you can grab what you want in a second instead of having to search through the whole suitcase. Make sure they're see-through and buy them at the five and dime.

• Make sure all liquids are transferred to plastic bottles (including perfumes). Aerosols can pop open in unpressurized baggage compartments.

• Best bets in fabric: leather (doesn't wrinkle or show dirt), knits, light wools.

• Travel light—that's essential. Separates can be interchanged for variety. Boots are classic and appealing in the fall and wintertime and sandals are light and comfortable for the summer. Avoid the twelve-inch heels unless you're modeling them.

• When you pack, make sure pockets are empty and belts are removed; they cause wrinkles like nothing else.

• Don't try to fold your clothes as small and as neatly as you can. Lay them out—as long as they'll go. Use the *length* of your suitcase; don't stack blouses, sweaters, dresses.

• Certain things like belts, socks and stockings roll better than fold and can be stuffed into corners. Generally, though, the flatter you pack, even soiled laundry as it accumulates (in a plastic bag, please), the more room you'll have.

PACKING SEQUENCE

1. Bagged shoes (separately please) go in the corners. They should not lie on top of anything that wrinkles.
2. Knits, heavy wools, sweaters, underwear go on the first layer.
3. Flimsy or soft dresses and sweaters go on top.
4. The most delicate fabrics of all go on the very top.

You arrive, and despite your packing acuity, everything is wrinkled? Turn on the hot water in the bathroom after hanging your clothes there: The steam will work wonders.

DON'T FORGET

• The adapter that allows you to plug in your hair dryer, curlers, and so forth in European outlets.
• Cold-water wool wash is great for laundering everything from wools to silks (yes, you *can* wash silks—carefully, *and* in cold water).

Dressing Truisms

Style in clothing means many things. Here are some of the things it means to me:

BE OPEN-MINDED. Many of us haven't moved a step in style since our mothers told us to be polite to the salesperson. We're so entrenched in the shopping rules of the past that our minds are closed to new ways of looking at style in the eighties. What's happened is that the fashion industry was forced to acknowledge the diversity, ingeniousness, and individuality of the American woman and new ways of shopping for and improvising outfits evolved. A delightful, witty, feminine, and still classic mélange of clothing can be found all contained in the one look you've come to understand is your best look. So, if you love trench coats, keep the style and rethink the color, perhaps. Instead of the basic tan, mauve, plum, cinnamon can be smashing! You love warm-up suits? Try them in stripes instead of solids. You can still wear your look (man-tailored or frilly or whatever), but you can alter it for interest. That's style.

THINK BALANCE. Style means that you don't have a whole lot going on in many places. Big earrings, for instance, call for very little other jewelry. "Decoration" in the summer may be nothing more than a wonderfully colored sandal to set off a white dress.

FABRICS SHOULDN'T PULL PUNCHES. Dressing with style almost always means using natural fabrics. Polyester masquerading as silk, plastic pretending to be leather, rayon lying about being cotton, are not stylish. Your style, no matter what its message is, should go for *real* and not artificial. Furthermore, synthetics tend to be uncomfortable. Polyester may not wrinkle in the summertime, but it also doesn't breathe and it's hot as Hades. Oh, every now and then you can get away with a polyester-*blend* blouse which, if manufactured well, is quite close to the real thing. A truly chic woman, however, would rather own a great Irish wool sweater than a phony-baloney fun fur. She'd opt for one fabulous silk blouse and tell you to keep the six rayon ones.

COLOR SHOULD BE RELEVANT. Earth-tone dressing calls for colors that are related to the earth. That's browns, yellows, soft reds—navy blue has very little to do with the earth and so it probably would look lousy with brown. Colors don't have to match, but they do have to complement in a relevant way. If you're wearing copper, you should pick up coppery glints in all accessories—a warm burgundy, a brown but never a white, for example. White has no relevance at all to copper. Blue-tone clothing—the purples, violets, pinks—have very little relevance to ruddy colors. Every now and then a fabric might allow for great contrast in color, but it still should make sense; in summer, when flowers bloom in reds and yellows and greens together, a summer cotton may look terrific in many bright colors. Winter velvet, though, would probably look tacky in many colors. Choosing color takes a certain kind of common sense. Your pocketbook doesn't have to match your shoes, but sense says it should be related in some way.

On the opposite tack, if you try to match everything, you turn out to look like a predesigned *set*. Matching everything has no authority, no class.

AVOID THE FAVORITE MOTHER-OF-THE-BRIDE COLOR. It's aqua. Avoid aqua at all costs. Never wear aqua even if you *are* the mother of the bride.

THE EMPTY-WALLET SYNDROME. It does take some money to dress in style, and I'd be patronizing if I said you could always shop at the five and dime. The five and dime, even large stores like Sears, can't produce clothing in true style because they produce in mass amounts. Woolworth's or Sears doesn't carry that one-in-a-million blouse, that dress that's sensational because a truly talented person put time and experience into its special creation. But if you *have* to go the mass-produced route and buy very inexpensive clothing because of a limited budget, do try to express your own style with one or two good and unusual items every time you wear something less than terrific. This means that if a cheap pair of summer cotton shorts from J. C. Penney is topped off with a super leather belt, the mediocrity of the shorts tends to go unnoticed. An inexpensive and simple black dress can look very rich if you wear one outstanding piece of gold jewelry. You can get away with twenty-dollar wool slacks if a finely detailed silk shirt plays along.

SIMPLIFY YOUR LIFE . . . by simplifying your closet. Give to the Girl Scouts or the Salvation Army anything you haven't worn in the last two years. You will never, believe me, wear it if you haven't worn it in that time. Get your closet pared down to the basic wardrobe of thirteen or so separates and two or three dresses, suits, and pairs of shoes that work together. Otherwise you end up standing in a stupor, staring at odds and ends that are never right. A closet, pared down to clothes that work together, lends itself to a stylish look.

WHEN YOUR OWN INITIALS ARE ENOUGH. On almost every level through life, the designer dictatorship knows how to reach the masses. In college, we wear school sweatshirts that say Yale or Syracuse. What this really says is: "I Belong. I Have a Group That Loves Me." When we wear eyeglasses with the designer initials emblazoned on the frame in little rhinestones, the message we want to send out is "I Belong to a Rich, Classy Group That Loves Me." What the rhinestones really say, though, is "I Have No Individual Style and I Have to Pay Someone Else to Lend Me His (or Hers)." Having wealth and personal success doesn't necessarily breed style, and that's surely true in the case of the rhinestone initials. Or jeans that say French things. Or pocketbooks that say GGGGGGGGGGGG. Look—I don't mind an occasional hidden G, somewhere unobtrusive, but splattering yourself with someone else's initials or idea of chic, identifying with hordes, is not my idea of style. Apparently, some of the designers who have made a fortune from initials are beginning to see this too. In fact, Louis Vuitton (master of the initial stamp since 1896) is coming out with a suitcase line *without* initials. LV knows overkill when he sees it.

I remember reading in a fashion magazine Ralph Lauren's idea of the "New Mode." The New Mode was supposed to capture the attention and the dollar of the American woman by putting forth the "American Look . . . clothing as personal and enduring as a handmade quilt." Lauren had the right marketing sense to appeal to everyone's notion of a handmade quilt—someone's grandma making the quilt just for her family. The only trouble was that Ralph Lauren's initials were splayed all over the clothing that was supposed to be so personal, so American "quilty." It's great marketing, lovely for Mr. and Mrs. Lauren, but it has nothing to do with style.

THINK TWICE ABOUT FURS. If you are not among those who won't wear furs from a conservationist viewpoint, think hard anyway before you race out to spend your last dime on a fluffy thing. Furs can be tricky. Persian lamb and even poorly styled mink can be aging—can draw you *down*. Fluffy, *big* furs can be flamboyant but can also look silly if you are short. The key word for fur is Simplicity. Furs should not be *fussy* but sleekly styled. They should *never* be fake. If you can't afford fur or are opposed to it, there's nothing more stunning than a good cloth or wool coat with simple lines to avoid bulk.

HOW DO I KNOW WHETHER TO BUY THE DRESS? You ask yourself:
- Do I already have it?
- Does it really fit?
- Does it say what I want it to say about me?
- Does it look spectacular—not just good?

You *do not* ask yourself:
- Will I love it next year? (Who cares?)
- Do I have shoes for it?
- Is it so cheap I don't really have to love it?
- Will it change my life? (It won't!)

Diana Vreeland's Advice

No one has so consistently been identified with style as Diana Vreeland—the grande dame of fashion. Truman Capote once said that Ms. Vreeland gave him the following wise words about developing a sense of style in dress. "Any woman could be chic or permanently presentable if she did the following: discover for herself the right maquillage [makeup], the correct coiffure, the cloth color that suits her best, and shoes in which she feels smartest and most comfortable. The important thing is: once having chosen this decor, one must never change it. Never."

She's absolutely right. Every woman should always stick with the style of dressing that is right for her. That doesn't mean she has to wear the same clothes all the time—only the same *kind* of clothes. As I said in the beginning of this chapter, you have to wear your *self*, and that doesn't really change through the years. Candice Bergen looks best in tailored clothing. "Even when I do try something a bit flashy or trendy," Candice says, "I'm always so relieved to return to classic clothes. They're really the looks that suit me."

So—it's your "look" I'm talking about. If your best look is classic, somehow you don't look terrific in sweetheart necklines. If your best look is in clothes that move with unaffected ease, you'll never look right in stiffened skirts. Style is particular, individual, and definite; within that style are myriads of choices.

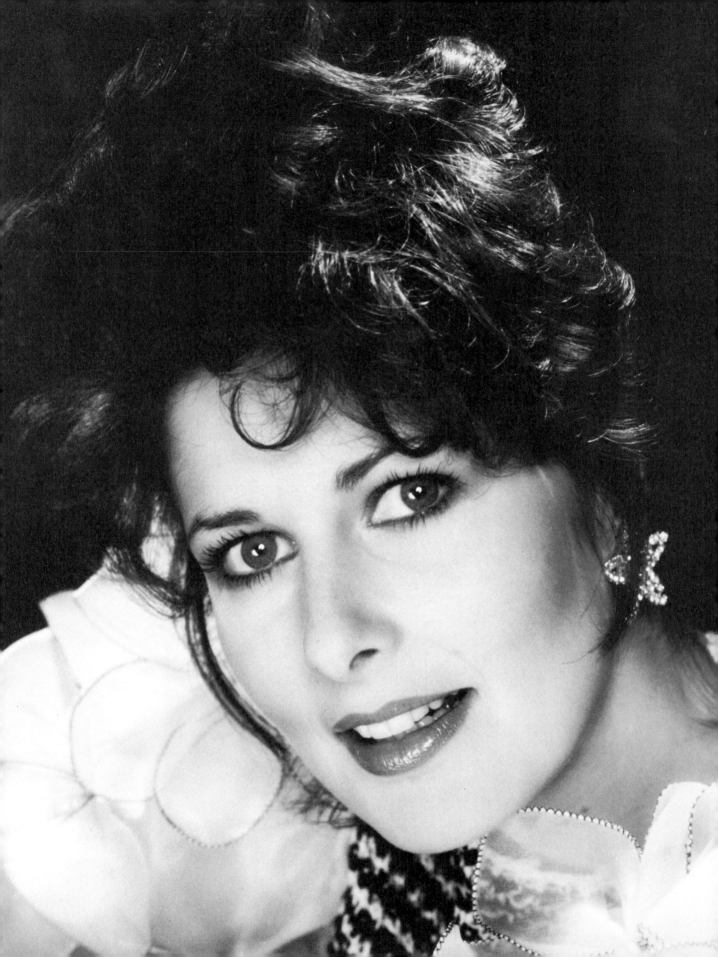

Chapter 2

MODEL FACES

*Y*OU don't have to be born with perfect features to have a model face, and if you look closely, you'll see that many of the most highly paid models in the industry are not necessarily natural beauties. What they have is the ability to put their best face forward. That means skin care and carefully applied makeup. Each is quite dependent on the other, because makeup is only as good as the skin on which you apply it. And make no mistake about it—there are special tricks that help enormously. I've been made up by some of the most skilled artists in the field; I've been experimenting with skin care and makeup for a whole lot of years, and I have many friends whose livelihood depends on looking fine. I'd like to share their beauty secrets with you. Remember one thing: As with fashion style, style of makeup and skin care differs from individual to individual. What works for me or for Cheryl Tiegs may not work for you. You have to experiment to find a makeup look that's right and a skin-care regimen that shows off your face to its prettiest. What follows are some of the things I've learned in the modeling game that just may be the tricks that can work wonders for the skin *you're* in and the face *you* make. Let's start with . . .

THE SKIN YOU WEAR

Keep It Moist!

In the beginning, there was—moisture. Moisture is the biggest secret ingredient in the creation of the smooth, pliant canvas on which you'll apply your makeup. I, and most of the models I know, moisturize in two ways:

FROM THE INSIDE OUT. Drink, drink, drink. When I'm not on a photography shoot and I'm reasonably near a bathroom, I drink from six to eight glasses of water a day. It not only gets rid of the solid, toxic junk in your system that eventually breaks out on your face, it helps enormously in weight reduction. Water is my one indispensable beauty treatment. I drink it, put it in the air I breathe, spray it on my skin and generally revel in it. When people think of a skin moisturizer, they think: oil. Wrong. Water is the only true moisturizer, and every skin product that says it rejuvenates faded, wrinkled, dry skin ought to have water in it as a major component. It's the only moisturizer that is readily absorbed by the skin; it softens, smooths, plumps out the lines caused by dryness and aging. While you can't avoid skin wrinkling from aging, you can avoid dryness, and it's important to water yourself internally as well as externally.

FROM THE OUTSIDE IN. The main purpose of moisturizing lotion is to seal the moisture into your skin. Therefore, the very best time to apply an oil-free moisturizer is right after your bath, when your skin is still beaded with water. After showering, or bathing, pat yourself reasonably (but not completely) dry; gently massage the moisturizer into your face and body. Use a moisturizer every night before bed and every morning before applying makeup. The morning application not only moisturizes but acts as a shield between your pores and your makeup. It also helps the foundation base to slide on evenly and smoothly. In between moisturizing treatments, and whenever I think of it during the day, I give my face a little spritz of Evian or mineral water from a tiny atomizer I carry around with me. Nothing like it for enlivening the facial tissues.

WATER IN THE AIR. Particularly in the winter when the steam heat is murderously drying to your face, you have to put some water back into the air. You can do this in two ways:

1. Place a pan of water on the radiator. As the steam works to heat and dry the atmosphere, the water will evaporate into the air—providing moisture for thirsty skin.

2. Sleep with a vaporizer. When you were little, your mother put a vaporizer in the room to ease your breathing when you had a cold. All it did was wet down the arid air. Wetting down the air is like the gift of lotion for a parched skin.

THE DEBIT SIDE OF WATER. Sometimes, if you are really conscientious about moisturizing, your face tends to have a bloated, puffy look in the morning from all the water-flushing inside and out. I find that sleeping slightly elevated, by placing a book under each of the bed's legs at the head, causes the excess water to drain nicely out of my facial tissues. It's a healthy way to sleep, anyway.

Keep It Clean!

Despite the fact that your mother told you dirt makes pimples, it doesn't. She also might have told you depressing things about eating fried foods and chocolate. Although eating all those oily substances doesn't do a whole lot for your shape, it really doesn't do much to sabotage your skin. What does do in your skin depends on the stage of life you're enjoying. During adolescence, the hormonal glands that zip up your sexuality also zip up the oil and sebum (a fatty secretion of the sebaceous glands) production. That increased oil not only tends to clog pores, it also traps bacteria on your skin. That's the way pimples, cysts, and other dermal ills are born. As we age, there are other skin destroyers that come into play; notable among them: the sun, drying soaps, birth-control pills, the slowed-up moisture retention qualities of the skin—and skin scurf. What's skin scurf? Simple. The skin is composed of several layers, and the outermost layer, the epidermis, replaces itself monthly. The used cells just flake off. At least it would be good if they flaked off, but what really happens is that some cells flake off and the others just sort of sit there, gathering in lines and making them look deeper than they really are, acting like plastic covers on pores and like gauze that clouds the healthy glow of good skin. Cleaning the skin means getting this outer layer of dead cells really *off*. Cleaning the skin also means taking off all makeup nightly. I've developed a kind of ritual for cleaning skin. Its most sterling virtue is its simplicity. My skin needs to be consistently good; no one wants to hear about your pimples when he's paying you big bucks to walk down that runway.

Five Minutes to Clean Skin

CLEAN

Every night of my life, I pat a soft, organic, nonperfumed cleanser, in either a liquid or a cream form, on my eyes and all over my face. I use a water-soluble product that doesn't leave a film on the skin, allow it to sit a minute which loosens the dirt, and then, with a sponge literally soaked full with warm water, I rinse off the cleanser (and makeup and dirt with it) from my face.

SCRUB AND MOISTURIZE

About twice a week I give myself a treatment with a honey-and-almond scrub that smells so good I feel like eating it. This removes the dead skin flakes from my skin. The tiny bits of almond act as a gentle abrasive, which scrubs away the skin flakes and the excess oil, and, what's more, adds tone and a healthy glow to the *look* of my skin. I apply the scrub to a clean, damp skin (everywhere but around the fragile eye area), massage it very gently in a circular motion for about ten or fifteen seconds, and remove it with the softest of cotton balls and then a whole lot of water splashed on my skin. After the scrub, I always apply moisturizer, which protects the new young skin I've just exposed.

All kinds of mild skin scrubs are available from skin-care counters in department stores or from skin-care experts (a trip to the latter might be a worthwhile thing to do).

Many of my associates in the business of beauty add another step to the skin-cleansing process, and that is applying a facial masque every once in a while. I hardly ever use masques because they seem to dry out my skin. However, because so many people swear by them, I offer the following information so you can make your own decision as to whether to add a weekly facial masque to your skin-cleansing regimen.

MASQUES

Masques are substances applied to the face that harden after a few minutes in varying degrees, depending upon their composition. When you remove a masque, your skin is supposed to react in different ways. A masque is supposed to tighten the skin, to stimulate, to deep clean, or to moisturize, depending upon its ingredients. What a masque *cannot* do—and I don't care who tells you otherwise—is remove wrinkles. A facial masque is soothing for some women, and it does provide a kind of sybaritic pleasure and relaxation as you lay there waiting for it to make magic. It's a good idea to put a thin film of moisturizer on your face under your masque to prevent the skin from drying out too much or from pulling as you remove the masque. There are wonderful-sounding variations of aloe, clay, collagen, honey, seaweed, and you-name-it masques, but, as I said, I hardly ever use them because they seem to dry out my skin. If you choose to use a masque that is supposed to deep clean by tightening and constricting pores, don't be discouraged if your face looks dreadful for a day or so after using it. The professional model knows that a cleansing masque that's worth the money you pay for it will push out impurities by tightening the skin around the pores; as a result, your face will show that something's happening by breaking out for a short while.

The only way to see if something works for you is to try it. Below are some masques that can be put together in your kitchen. They are different kinds of masques to be used for different purposes. Before you spend a whole lot of money on a commercial product, perhaps you would like to experiment (and maybe decide to keep) one of these:

THE CLAY MUDPACK. This mask is for deep cleansing. Ask your druggist for a colloidal kaolin (it's the substance found in almost all clay masques) and mix half a cup with two teaspoons of tincture of benzoin and enough distilled water to make a loose paste. Smear it on your face and allow it to harden; after about ten minutes, rinse with a warm, wet cloth and see if you feel that facial oil and dirt have been drawn out.

THE OATMEAL MASQUE. This mask seems to be helpful in removing flaky skin and surface blackheads because oatmeal has a rough, exfoliating quality. Moisten a cup of raw oatmeal with enough water to make a paste. Let it dry; massage it off gently after about ten minutes and rinse your face with warm water.

THE HONEY AND ALMOND MASQUE. This is primarily a face softener rather than a cleanser. Heat two tablespoons of almond oil in two tablespoons of fresh honey and allow to cool to a comfortable temperature. Apply it to your face, allow it to remain for about fifteen minutes, and then remove with a warm cloth. Follow with a moisturizer.

THE WHIPPED EGG MASQUE. Whip an egg yolk with a drop of oil added, apply it to your face and allow it to dry. Whip the white of the egg to a froth, apply it to your face over the yolk and allow it to remain for about ten minutes. Remove it with a warm, wet, soft cloth. This masque, when followed with a moisturizer, seems to soften lines by cleansing the accumulated dead skin cells from them.

WARNING: Scented masques and masques with heavy doses of astringents added tend to irritate sensitive skin. It's a good idea to follow each masque with a gentle moisturizer.

The Skin Drink That's Better than a Malted

In every profession, there are tricks of the trade, and one of the best ones I know is the collagen drink. You don't drink it with your mouth—your skin drinks it by absorption. Collagen is a protein substance found in the body's connective tissues that provides the skin with its elasticity. As you age, the skin loses some of its collagen—the prime cause of skin sag, wrinkling, and lining. Collagen exists in the dermis, the layer of skin that's below the epidermis, or surface skin. Many scientists say that substances applied to the epidermis (lotions, potions, creams, and so on) cannot be absorbed into the second layer, the dermis. I don't buy that argument for a moment. I'm not a doctor, and I don't know the scientific reasoning behind absorption, but I know that my skin has never looked and felt as good in my life as it has since I started applying a clear collagen moisture lotion twice daily. My skin feels softer and more resilient—it is definitely more moist. Many skin lotions have collagen ingredients added, and I suggest you give one a try or go to a health-food store or a skin-care expert to find a product that's composed almost totally of collagen. No one has ever said it can hurt you—and I, and many other top models, literally swear by its benefits.

Some "Fast Takes" on Skin

HOW TO WINTERIZE YOUR SKIN

• Never emerge into the wind, sleet, glare, snow, or ice without a moisturizing cream. Makeup is a great protector also.

• Apply a special moisturizing cream around the eyes, a particularly sensitive area; eye creams are lighter than regular facial creams.

• If you *have* to use soap to feel clean, try a clear, transparent soap like Pears or Neutrogena or a super-fatted one like Dove. Avoid detergent, deodorant, and medicated soaps, which often contain abrasive chemicals. I never could understand medicated soaps anyway—you rinse them off and right down the drain before they can do any good with their medicine. I far prefer mild cleansing lotions or creams to soaps—any soaps.

HOW TO SUMMER-PROOF YOUR SKIN

• Use a light foundation base at all times—for sun protection.

• At the beach, use a sun block with a protective factor (the highest SPF is fifteen and gives the most protection, depending on your skin's needs).

• Cleanse more often. That means using a very mild exfoliating cream occasionally to rid the skin of surface flakes and dirt.

• If you use an oil-based moisturizer (you really shouldn't, anyway), consider changing it, at least for the summer. Heat speeds up metabolism and in so doing gives a booster to oil glands. Result? More oil production.

• Take the sun in small doses. A little glow is just as healthy *looking* as a massive suntan and much better for your skin.

The Face You Make

Makeup is the most extraordinary invention since the wheel and, actually, I think it's been around a lot longer. All through the ages women have thought of putting color on their faces to make themselves prettier. Cave woman painted her face with berry juice. Nefertiti used kohl; lovely Grecian ladies thought white chalk made their classic profiles more classic, and they also were not beyond dabbing a bit of barley powder on their Greek pimples to make them a tad less classic. American Indians used war paint to help them win battles and American women (and almost all other women) use another kind of war paint to fight other kinds of battles. It seems battles are won more easily when people are impressed with the way you look. And makeup does change the way you look—for better and, sometimes, for a lot worse . . . if you're not skilled.

I love makeup. Sometimes, I wake up in the morning absolutely beset with problems I have to work out before the day's end. My face looks it, too. And then I go to a photography session, and a makeup artist starts reconstructing my face with glorious color. Where my eyes are puffy from lack of sleep, he dabs on concealer. Where my skin is pale from lack of air or exercise, he makes it blush with the most wondrous color. Where my bones have gotten lost in pudge because my dieting has been on the blink, he sculpts out bones with contour. He takes what I think are nice eyes and makes them magnificent with a dab here, a line there. Before I know it, I'm ready to put on—and do justice to—a wonderful gown. And, what's more important, because I feel I look pretty, I also feel I can cope with anything. The morning's problems seem to pale, I think straighter, stand straighter, and am generally a nicer person not only to look at but to speak with. Because of something as mundane as makeup. Not so mundane, after all.

A Model Makeup

You really don't need a hundred different products and tools. Often your fingers are the best makeup tool of all. What you do need for a professional makeup are the *right* tools, a few good products, and the knowledge of what each thing does. The beauty business is big business, and often the same products are called different names to hype them up. For instance: fresheners, toners, astringents, and clarifying lotions—would you believe? *All the same.* They are liquids applied to the skin to remove accumulated oils and dirt, give a natural glow by tightening pores (I'm not so sure they can really do that) or restore the natural acid mantle of the skin, which may be changed by alkaline substances like certain soaps and lotions. The only difference in all these products is that some contain more alcohol than others; if it's called an astringent, it probably has the most alcohol and if it's called a freshener, it probably has little or no alcohol and mostly water. I know women who proudly own fresheners, toners, astringents, and clarifying lotions and don't know that they're wasting a whole lot of money on the same thing with a different title. Foundations are bases also. Cleansing lotions and creams are the same thing except one is liquid, the other more solid. Highlighters, gleamers, and glows are the same product. They play up an area by changing the color or texture somewhat. Okay—with all these babies from a Madison Avenue copywriter, where do you start to get the very best, and also simplest, model makeup?

First you set the stage. Take a look at your makeup collection. *Throw out:*
  • whatever you haven't used this year (you won't use it, period);
  • whatever you can't identify;

- whatever you've inherited from someone else with different coloring (it'll look ghastly on you);
- whatever smells funny.

Presumably you now have a freshened, empty-ish makeup collection. What do you get for it?

The Basic Makeup Tools

1. *Four Good, Fat Sable Brushes* (a smaller one for eye shadow, one for contour, one for eye liner, one for powder and blusher). Don't stint here and buy cheap brushes; sable ones will last forever (well, almost).
2. *One Eyelash Curler.*
3. *One Tweezers.*
4. *One Box of Cotton Swabs* (for applying concealer, dotting on makeup, removing smudges).
5. *Small Applicators* with foam tips for eye shadows.
6. *One Lip Brush* (for applying color and/or gloss to the mouth).

The Basic Makeup

1. *The Moisturizer.* This helps your foundation glide on and last longer.
2. *Three to Four Lipsticks.* All you ever really need is a soft plum or burgundy to match your natural lips. You can temper the look of each lipstick with lip gloss in red, bronze, pink, or natural to blend with your outfit. Many lipsticks in a makeup collection tend to dry out, be unused, and serve as clutter.
3. *One Foundation Base* that matches (as close as you can get it) your own skin. Liquid foundation that's water (not oil) based is best for those with good skin, and cream is best for those who need more coverage.
4. *Two or Three Powder Blushers* in a soft rosy tone (evening blushers can have a slight shine).
5. *One Powder Contour* in a rust or brownish shade.
6. *One Cream Rouge* in a soft red, coral, or pink—depending on what looks best on you.
7. *One Concealer.*
8. *One Box of Translucent Powder.*
9. *Three or Four Eye Shadows.*
10. *Artificial Lashes.* If you must wear them, wear individual lashes, which look far more natural than the whole strip—place on with tweezers as close to the lash line as possible.

11. *One Brow Crayon* that matches your natural brows and is kept very sharp.
12. *One Lip-liner Pencil* in a color that picks up the tone of your natural lips.
13. *One Black Mascara Wand.*
14. *Highlighter.* This is a gel with a bit of iridescent powder added to it. A stroke or two on cheekbones or brows gives your face a special glow for evening.
15. *One Dark Eye Shadow Color* in black or brown to use as eye liner when wet (applied with a tiny, pointed brush).

Okay, the stage is set. Now you make your play.

Here are the easy steps to follow for a glowing, fabulous makeup. I've broken them down to two special looks: one is the Daytime Look and the other is the Killer Makeup—when you really want to knock them dead!

The Daytime Look—Eight Steps to Dynamite!

1. START WITH A CLEAN FACE, naturally. *Nothing's* going to look spectacular (or even passable) with last night's oil peeking through. Now, put on a very thin layer of moisturizer and softly massage it onto your face.

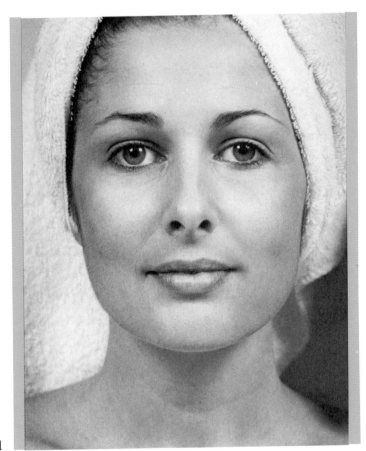

1

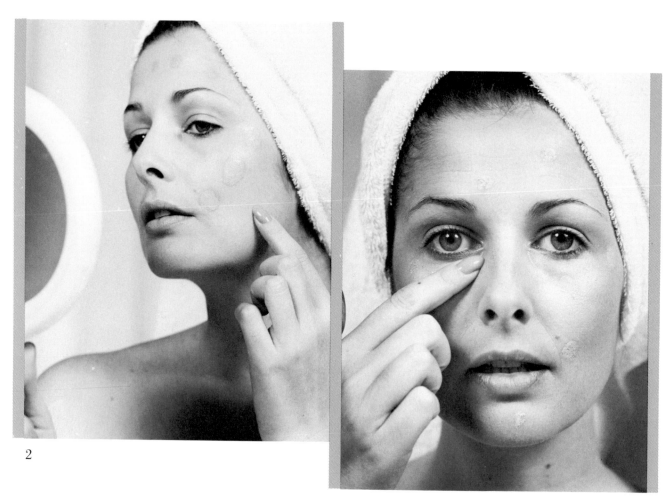

2

3

2. *DOT ON YOUR MAKEUP BASE* and blend it softly all over your face, including your lips. The base should be in a shade that's equal to your natural skin tone; a darker base stains imperfections and makes them more obvious. Foundation base is not for adding color to the face at all. Its purpose is to even out the pigment of the skin and provide an even canvas for the color (the rouge, blusher, lipstick, and so on).

3. *HERE COMES THE DISAPPEARING ACT!* Dot on and then blend (with your fingertips) some concealing liquid on any dark spots, spidery vessels, blemishes, under-eye dark lines.

TIP: For those morning puffy eyes, dot the concealer just on the line of demarcation *under* the puffiness. If you put the concealer on the whole puff, it will highlight it instead of conceal it.

Don't blend to the point where the blemish or line shows through again: Practice and a subtle touch will allow you to cover. Use a liquid concealer, by the way, because cream, cake, and pencil tend to congeal.

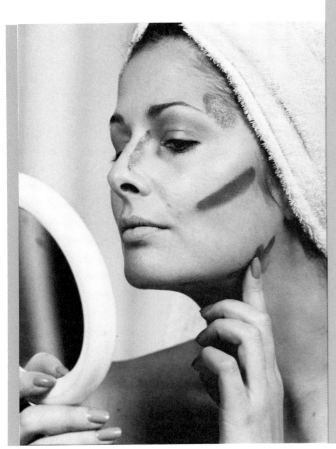

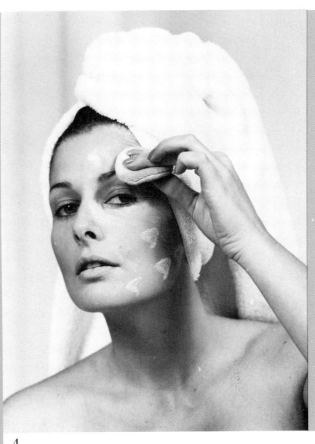

4

4. *TIME FOR THE CONTOUR:* If you are less than totally satisfied with your facial bone structure, you need a *little* contour shading (you can go heavier in the Killer Makeup which follows). Contour goes *under* the cheekbone. Feel your face and pay attention to the hollow that's under the cheekbone; you'll discover where to brush on the rusty-brown powder—*in* the hollow and *out* from the middle of the cheek hollow to the hairline in an upward slanting direction. The purpose of contouring is to add interest to your face by sculpting out bones; go lightly for daylight use, blend well into the foundation to avoid a stripey look and don't end before the hairline—go right into it. Contour can be lightly brushed down the sides of a wide nose and on the underside of a chin to "paint out" skin sag or double chins as best as possible. Make sure you blend, blend, blend with your brush and with translucent powder over all. Lightly powdering *many* times during makeup application ensures a professional look.

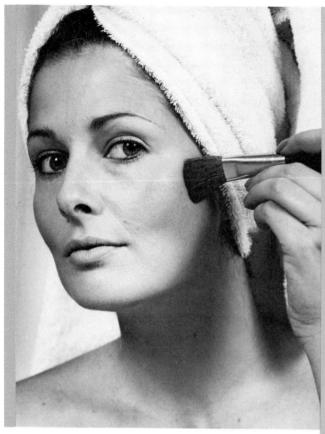

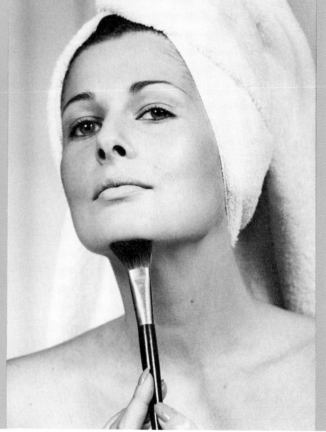

5

5. *TIME FOR THE CHEEK COLOR!* A light cream rouge spotted *onto* the cheek bone (above and following the contour line) and well blended adds life to your face. Rouge should never be in a screaming color but should simulate a natural blush. I love pinky, not red, tones, for me anyway, and my makeup color password is always *soft*. A little powder blusher in the same shade dusted with a fat sable brush over the rouge sets it. Dust a little blusher on the chin and forehead also—even on the tip of the nose. That's a natural look—when you blush, color comes into your face in many places.

6. *TIME FOR THE EYES!* Even when I'm in a desperate hurry and have time for only the most minimal of makeup, eyes have priority.
    • *Eye Shadows Come First.* You must experiment with many powder shadows to achieve pretty looks, but always with one principle in mind:

lightness points out—darkness conceals. If you have, for instance, a puffy eyelid or an eyelid that droops, you will want to put your darkest shadows on the lid. They will then be gently blended into a lighter shadow applied directly under the brow to exaggerate the width and space of the eye and draw attention away from that puffy lid. A look I like is a soft shadow in a dusky brown shade on the lid, blended up and into a golden or pinky shade that softly covers the eye-bone area and goes up to the brow. If you shadow more deeply at the corners of the eye (at the crease), you achieve a terrific Oriental-type look. A soft teal or deeper blue or purple on the lids looks wonderful when blended into a pink or gold that highlights the brow bone. Eye shadow should not match the eye but contrast and draw attention to it. However, you can pick up a fleck of color that's in your eye or clothing when you choose shadow. Eye shadow should not be in any other form but powder. Creams congeal in the creases giving a not-so-terrific look of gloppiness.

• *I Curl My Lashes* with a metal lash curler after I apply the shadows, taking care to open the curler before removing it from the lashes (along with two thousand lashes).

• *The Liner Comes Next.* I use an old-fashioned technique for liner because I think it looks more subtle than a pencil or a liquid liner. I dip a soft brush in water and then in a charcoal gray or sable brown eye shadow powder. I get enough color on the brush to give an eyelash line that's much softer than the kind you get from a hard pencil or liquid liner. I line *on* and directly *beneath* the lower eyelash line and *on* and directly *above* the upper lash line. There should never be a space between your lash line and the line which you draw on.

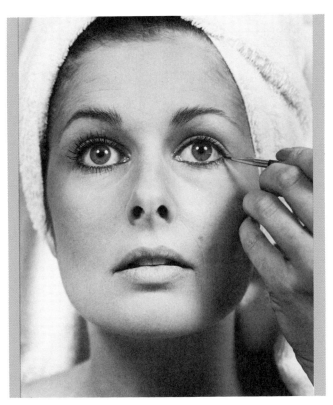

6

• *After the Liner Dries*, I rub it gently with a sponge brush to blend it. There's nothing worse than an artificially hard line. Then I sweep on the thickest, blackest mascara (everyone, no matter what color lashes, should wear black mascara), being careful not to clump my lashes. Two or three coats of mascara, with each coat drying in between, are better than one thick coat.

• *Deal with Your Brows* as the next step. You will have plucked any stray hairs from your brows, following their natural line, the day before. (If you do it right before your makeup, you may have to contend with a reddened puffy eyebrow area.) But what if you have naked spots in your brow line, or if your brows are too short? You'll need to feather them in with the most natural, hairlike lines, and to do this, you'll use a pencil in your own brow color that's been sharpened to the absolutely sharpest point. Now here's a real model's trick: Brush your browns *down* with an old soft toothbrush before you feather in a single line. Feather in sparse areas when your brows are brushed down, *then* cover those lines as you gently sweep the brow back up. The brow line

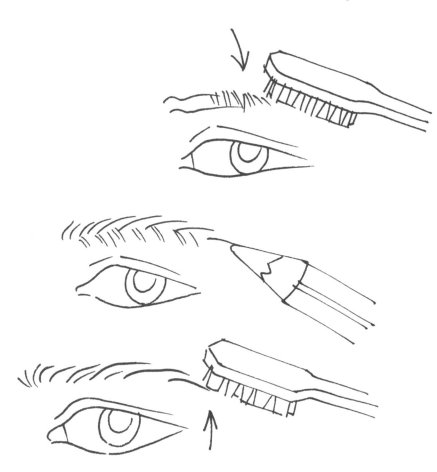

will look as natural as can be with your own brow hairs covering most of the pencil lines. The absolute worst look in the world is a brow that's been drawn on in a single dark line or a brow that's been thickened with inky black pencil. The purpose of "cleaning out" stray or thickly grown brow hair is to create space between your brows and the eyes. That gives you room for work with color to add depth, width, and interest to your eyes.

7. *A LIGHT DUSTING OF TRANSPARENT COLORLESS POWDER* comes on next, over everything except your eyes. Your lips should have a layer of foundation on them from the very beginning of the makeup, and now you dust lightly over your lips with powder to prepare for the lip color. (Foundation evens out the lip color so that lipstick goes on evenly. The powder helps the lipstick to stay on.)

8. *THE MOUTH IS LAST*. I always line my lips with lip liner. That gives you cleanly defined and wonderful lips and also prevents the lipstick from "bleeding"

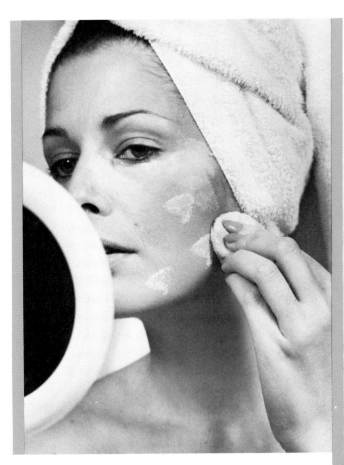

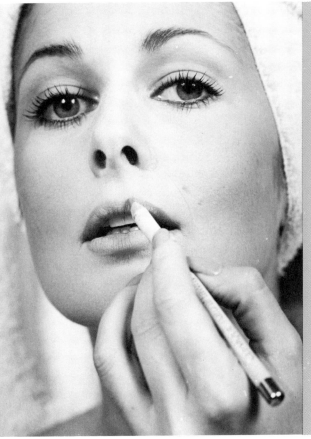

into the tiny little lines that eventually develop around the lips. *Be sure* to take your little finger and blend the lip line softly down into your lips after you've drawn it. A sharply outlined mouth always looks as if you've just eaten a chocolate cupcake.

Your lipstick should blend with your skin tone and should never clash with your clothing. That means if you have tons of purple in your natural lips, common sense dictates staying away from ruby red shades. Red lipstick looks disconcerting, to say the least, with violet dresses. Subtle lip color is always more sensual than garish blasts of color. Lipstick should be applied with a brush onto the outlined lips. For an irresistible transparent berrylike glow, apply lipstick and then apply a touch of nongluey lip gloss. Don't cake on a *lot* of lipstick; lip color should never be *thick* because that will make it bleed and, worse, make it creep onto your teeth. Nothing tackier.

Your makeup is finished (see Daytime Look makeup in "Personal Style" insert)! After you've practiced a bit, the whole thing shouldn't take more than ten or fifteen minutes. Anyone who spends an hour putting on day makeup is either a klutz or putting on too much makeup. Check the *whole* effect carefully, and add or delete where necessary. The *only* place to check, in the daytime, is in natural light. Beauty in the real world does not depend on a perfect nose or high cheekbones. It depends on makeup skill. All the "natural" beauties know that. They wear more makeup than anyone—very artfully applied. You can be sure of that.

The Killer Makeup!

What's the Killer Makeup? It's almost always an evening makeup for an occasion where it's absolutely necessary that you look your most extravagant *gorgeous!* It follows the same basic outline as the Daytime Look makeup, but almost everything is a little more dramatic. In addition, there are a few *additions* to the Killer Makeup that should be nonexistent in a daytime makeup. Killer makeups should be savored like fine wines and employed only now and then. For instance, you wouldn't wear your killer makeup to a movie. It would be wasted and probably not even appreciated. Killer makeups are created for
- when you get to meet the Queen;
- when you get to meet that fabulous new man, starting off your relationship with a Broadway opening or a night at the opera;
- when you're going to the "beautiful people" cocktail party;
- when you're hosting the most stylish dinner party in town;
- when you're planning a romantic, at-home rendezvous just for the two of you.

Okay—Killer Makeup is dependent on high drama, not a heavy-handed, gloppy, *thick* makeup. Therefore, the amount of foundation stays the same, but the color that's added to it is intensified. To be specific:

• The contour (Step Four of daytime makeup) becomes more deeply applied. You will still have to blend, of course—otherwise you'll have cheek stripes—but you can brush on more color, which will more deeply delineate your bone structure. To keep everything balanced, you will then add a bit more color to the cheeks in the form of blusher and rouge, always meticulously blending so the effect is dramatic but soft—*very unlike* the Streetwalker Effect and *very like* the Glamour Effect.

• Extraordinary eye effects are what Killer Makeup relies on heavily. You can line the *insides* of your lash lines (the mushy part) with an eye-liner pencil for eyes that call out: "Look at me!" Caution: Line the insides only *if* your eyes are reasonably large; small eyes get closed in with this technique. You can brush on a subtle gold glow of highlighting powder on the brow bone for added glamour. Killer eye shadow is often an intensification of daytime shadow. Experiment with color, keeping the *light brings out, dark conceals* theory in mind. Just remember: *Never match* your iris color to shadow. It will *de*emphasize the eye.

Killer eye makeup often employs false eyelashes. I'll tell you something about false eyelashes: They can either look tacky or very glamorous. If you go for the fringed look, take my advice: Even though it takes longer, cut the strip of eyelash into individual lashes and apply them with Duo Eyelash Adhesive *one at a time*. Put them on from the middle of the lash line out to the outside corner— never on the inner corner of the lash line, which looks blatantly false. You can buy individualized lashes at drugstores or makeup departments. They're sold in groups of longer and shorter lashes, or you can cut a full-size lash into individual lashes. Be sure your eyes are made up and you have applied mascara. The lashes are applied with a tweezer right on top of your own lashes (not on the lid). They're removed by holding a warm, wet cloth or cotton pad to the eye for a few moments which loosens them; then, dipping a cotton swab into the lash remover that comes with most artificial lashes, you gently pat the lash with the cotton swab, which eventually removes it. Never pull off artificial lashes. See finished Killer Makeup in "Personal Style" insert.

TIP: False lashes come in a synthetic material and in a human-hair lash. Even if you have to spend a little more, go for the human-hair lash; the other is artificial looking.

ANOTHER TIP: Never wear false lashes that are more than a millimeter longer than your own lashes. That looks gauche and just unbelievable. Here are some further killer suggestions:

THE CHEEKBONES. Pearlized or frosted powder can look fantastic when just a smidgen's worth is added to the very tip of the cheekbone; a face with a matte finish (every face should have a matte finish if the face is more than eleven years old) looks stunning with a touch of glow to call attention to only one spot—at night only, never in the daylight.

THE LIPS. A nice Killer touch to lips is a smudge of a bit of gold glittery powder right in the center of the lower lip. Talk about sensuality . . .

THE BODY. If you know you're going to be wearing a strapless or a very open or low-cut neckline, try a tinted body lotion that's for sale at most makeup counters. (Stage Ten, Diane Von Fürstenberg and Madeleine Mono are some of the manufacturers that carry body highlighter.) A little goes a long way, but it gives a fantastic effect—especially under night lights.

CAUTION: Shimmering may be fun for disco-type parties, but may be very inappropriate for a more elegant sedate affair. Use your judgment.

SPOTLIGHT FOR A TAN. If you have a golden tan, a bronzelike *gel*, applied (after a very light foundation base) on the cheekbones gives a real glow to the face.

The Emergency Makeup

Some days are pretty tight. Also some nights. When you have absolutely no time for a careful daytime makeup—when you could not possibly do justice to a Killer nighttime makeup, what's the least you can get away with? It's the emergency makeup and it's this:

1. A foundation—just dotted on in the crucial spots and blended.
2. A dash of blusher.
3. A curl of lashes and a sweep of mascara.
4. A dusting of powder on the nose.
5. A dollop of lip gloss on softly outlined lips.

Go ahead, face the world—you look just fine!

BEAUTY TIPS

Keep It On (How to Make Makeup Last Longer)

EYES

• If you powder the lid with a white eye shadow before you put on your color shadow, the color won't swim away in an hour.

• If you sprinkle a bit of translucent powder on your finger or a mascara brush and coat (lightly) your lashes before applying mascara, it'll have far more staying power.

• If you allow the first coat of mascara to dry before adding a second coat, the mascara will last much longer.

LIPS

• As has been mentioned, coat your lips with foundation to even out the color before applying lipstick. Then lightly powder with translucent powder. Outline lips with lip liner, apply lipstick with lip brush, blot, lightly powder again, and apply the final coat of lipstick and/or gloss.

FACE

• Powder blushers have much longer lasting power than cream ones.

• Lightly powder the face with a fat brush and translucent powder after applying the foundation base and after the blusher and contour.

Keep It Clean

• Wash your makeup brushes every few days in the top shelf of the dishwasher (but take them out before the dry cycle). Let them air dry.

• Wet cotton swabs make handy removers; you get a clean one every time.

• If someone wants to borrow your eye makeup, say no. If someone wants to borrow your lipstick, say no. The quickest route to eye and mouth infections is saying yes.

• *Never* (argh) spit in powdered makeup to wet it.

Keep It Easy

• For the easiest way to the smudged look, rub a small brush several times across your eye-lining pencil, then glide the brush along your lash line.

• The easiest way to put dynamic color on the wet ledge of the lower lid is to gently pull down the skin under the lid to expose more ledge and then *slide* (don't dab or press) the pencil along the rim.

Keep It Comfortable

The eyes are probably the most sensitive part of you, and fatigue, water retention, and makeup reactions can make them irritated or puffy. Here are some fast tips that every model knows will give her fast relief:

FOR EYE PUFFINESS. Cooled tea bags (the cheaper the better because cheap tea has more tannic acid) placed on your eyes for ten minutes reduces puffiness.

FOR REDNESS OR ITCHINESS. Chilled raw potato or cucumber slices on your eyelids relieve itchy reddened eyes.

FOR FATIGUE. Cotton balls soaked in cold milk do wonders when placed on the eyes for ten or fifteen minutes.

FOR REMOVING THAT SPECK OF DUST OR EYELASH. Simply squeeze an eye-wash solution into the eye right from the bottle or from an eye cup. Blink several times. *Carefully* wipe the object from the eye with a wet cotton swab.

Models' Tricks of the Trade

If there's one thing models know about, it's making pretty faces. Here are some skin and makeup "in" tips from my colleagues, eleven of the most exquisite women in the world—the Million-Dollar Models.

CARMEN

"Skin secret? For me it's vitamin E. As I've aged, my skin has gotten extremely dry and I know how to soften it! I just open up a vitamin E capsule, dump the liquid contents into my nightly bath water, and my skin, after forty, is the same as it was at twenty. Some days, to give my face a rest, I don't wear any makeup at all—just a little mineral oil for moisture.

"Makeup secret? I dye my eyelashes. What a great invention for those of us who hate and/or are allergic to mascara. It costs about twenty dollars, lasts for about a month. After they're dyed, I put a little Elizabeth Arden Eight-Hour Cream, mineral oil, or that vitamin E liquid on the eyelash tips to keep them moist and gleaming. Be careful you don't confuse vitamin E with vitamin A, which is fish oil—it takes a month to get the smell out."

CHRISTIE BRINKLEY

"Water is my magic. I put a steam room in my shower and whenever I turn it on, I feel the moisture just going back into my skin. I drink at least eight glasses of water a day and sleep with a vaporizer in my room.

"Makeup trick? It's lighting. I always put on my makeup, in the daytime, by a window in the light in which it will be seen. If anything is too sharp, I mute it with some translucent powder which blends subtly."

KIM ALEXIS

"My trick is for natural blondes. A little lemon juice mixed with coconut oil and a drop of peroxide, sprayed on the hair before sitting in the sun, makes blond hair as sunny as a Caribbean day. Lemon juice is a natural bleach, but most hairdressers won't divulge that information." (Note from me, Cristina: Use a good moisturizing rinse after your lemon juice treatment because lemon is a strong astringent and will dry out your hair if you don't compensate for it.)

"Also, I have blue-gray eyes, but I never match my shadow to them. Instead, I'll often put a little pink blusher on my lids which kind of opens up my eyes— makes them look larger. Eye liner is drawn around the entire rim of my eye and I make sure to smudge it so it doesn't look hard. If you match your eye color, attention is drawn *away* from the eyes and to the eye shadow."

CARRIE NYGREN

"A wonderful model's trick for red and puffy eyes—the kind you get after a good cry: massage ice cubes around the eye and the puffiness disappears in twenty minutes.

"I always curl my lashes, put subtle gray and brown shadows on in the winter and blue ones that make my eyes stand out in the summer, and I *love* to use my black mascara. I'm from Sweden, and we know that saunas are great for skin. After the sauna, very important, use an alcohol astringent to close the opened pores."

ANETTE STAI

"I use the cheapest products I can find and they're just as good as the high-priced brands. Lubriderm (you can buy it in the drugstore) is my favorite cleanser; Doak Pharmacal Formula 405 is my favorite moisturizer, and Cetaphil is my all-time best heavy makeup remover. And vitamins—whenever I travel, I take a double dosage of vitamin C. The B-complex vitamins never fail to give me better skin and extra strength—especially around my period."

CAROL ALT

"Eight-Hour Cream right under my eyes! The cream picks up light and pulls attention to the eyes. I even dab a bit of it over my lipstick for a highlighting effect."

SHEILA JOHNSON

"Very few black women realize that our skin has many reddish and blue tints to it. Picking up one of those colors in makeup looks gorgeous! I love reddish-coral blushers (never orange!) and grays, turquoises, and dark blues on my eyelids look very glamorous, very elegant."

RENÉE RUSSO

"Products that are perfume-free! Clinique is terrific."

JANICE DICKINSON

"Beauty comes from within. Instead of piling pounds of glop on your face, buy yourself a few great records and let your face dance with the music. Then you'll be beautiful. For hair and body vitality, end each shower with a two-minute huffing and puffing in a cold-water rinse, singing 'Rhinestone Cowboy' at the top of your lungs!"

NANCY DONAHUE

"I don't have a distinct lid on my eyes and they can tend to look hooded and indistinct. So I *create* a lid by putting a darker eye-shadow powder in the crease of the eye, a lighter color under my brow and another lighter color on the lid, and blend the colors into each other so you don't know where one starts and the other leaves off. Purply eye liner inside the lower lash line and a smudgy line of dark green shadow right under makes the whites of my eyes much whiter and 'opens' them, also."

EVA VORHEES

"Albolene. The whole secret to good skin is *taking off* the makeup."

Model Travel Tips

Sometimes a model is asked to fly eight hours and step off the plane and onto a runway. We've learned some tricks to thwart the beauty-damaging effects of altitudes and atmosphere changes.

• If you're planning to fly, moisturize your skin before, during, and after the flight. Nothing like being over the clouds to dry you out like a prune.

• Ask your doctor to recommend extra vitamins; nothing like them to make up for the changes in diet, atmosphere, and water.

• Ask for a bulkhead seat or an aisle seat or a seat by an exit door. They traditionally give the most room to stretch and keep the blood circulating. Ask your flight attendant for some warm socks as you remove your shoes while in the air; it's great for the circulation to rotate your toes (you might even throw a pair of warm socks in your purse for that reason).

• Drink a lot of water (fresh or mineral) while traveling in the air to replenish the moisture lost from lack of humidity.

• If you've got to be pretty perky in just hours after arrival, consider taking an antihistamine which will induce drowsiness and a snooze on the airplane.

• Never use the night shades the airlines sometimes give out. They prevent the eyes from blinking (which goes on even during sleep). Water accumulates and bags and circles are the result when you awake.

• Eat less in flight because pressure changes can cause indigestion.

• Don't have dental work performed less than twelve hours before you board the plane. Recent drilling or periodontic or root canal work at increased altitudes can expand and make you cry with pain.

The Thank-Goodness-It's-Been-Invented-Panacea

IT'S COSMETIC SURGERY!

And what happens if you've exhausted every makeup trick, every Revlon color, ever Killer Makeup device, and you still *hate-the-way-the-eyelid-puffs look!* I think that true style decrees that you take advantage of the miracles of science.

Where is it written that cosmetic surgery is immoral or vain? It's not even fattening. Being a stoic is not at all an example of living a life with panache—*unless* you really can't do anything about the thing that troubles you. (Then being a stoic is sensible.) Much better than stoicism is saving your pennies to find the very best and most highly recommended plastic surgeon in the world and have him . . .

- straighten your nose
- lift your left breast
- smooth wrinkles
- eliminate the eyelid puff
- banish the bags

or, as your mother used to say, "make it better." I'm not saying that it's terrific to run to a surgeon every time a wrinkle shows up. All I'm saying is that people used to die before penicillin was invented, used to be hot in the desert before air conditioning was invented, and *some* people used to look prematurely old before plastic surgey was invented. Style often depends on intelligently seizing options, and in these 1980s, we do have the option of safe, relatively comfortable plastic surgery. Once reserved for the rich and famous to indulge in secretly, cosmetic surgery is now a real possibility for anyone who wakes up in the morning hating her face. Whether we like it or not, if we're honest, we have to admit that looking good gives one renewed possibilities, both emotionally and actually.

Plastic surgery is not for everyone; if you don't mind the hooked nose, sags, bags and assorted crevices of years—terrific! *But if you do*, don't waste another minute feeling guilty because you care about your appearance in this way. Besides actual facial reconstruction, all kinds of procedures are available today including collagen injections to "plump up" skin depressions. Silicon injections, also used by some physicians to plump up skin, can have ghastly side effects, including scarring and discoloration and lumping, because silicon is a synthetic and often rejected by body tissues. Electrocautery is a process where tiny, broken capillaries (red spider lines) are removed from the skin surface and tiny lines and fine wrinkles can even be "shaved" off the skin's surface by yet another process. It's all expensive, and you can't very well attempt to return a face lift or a nose job if you hate it, as you can return a dress, but if you find the best doctor available, you have a very good chance of enhancing the thing you like least about your physical appearance. That "if" is a big one: Only a fool would try to find a bargain doctor. Get the one that comes most highly qualified and recommended.

HERE'S A CAUTION: The thing you cannot change with plastic surgery is your life, your essential self. You're still the same *you* with the same fears and the same promise—with maybe a nicer chin. So far, so good with *me* and my face and my body, but I'm telling you right now, I'm not going to live with fat eye puffs if I don't have to, even though I know my husband and kids will love me—puffs or no puffs. Why not? If I care enough about looking good to wear lipstick and mascara, I'd be lying if I said I loved the puffs.

Let me try to sum up what I've been saying in this section. Like the famous Levy's bread slogan, "You don't have to be Jewish to like Levy's," you definitely don't have to be born beautiful to have style. You don't even have to be beautiful to have beauty—if you know the makeup tricks. Both style and beauty are often *impressions* one gets from the essence of a woman: the wit and charm of her conversation, the clarity of her eyes (maybe enhanced with some shadow), her total presence. Style, in the long run, is a dizzying, glamorous aura you build about yourself, and the way your lipstick is applied and the way your mascara is coated on has less to do with style than the total look. I have seen women who have longish noses, thickened waists, far less than fabulous eyes and yet men fall at their feet and proclaim their extraordinary beauty—and *mean* it. Their clothes may come from a catalog and yet other women use them as style archetypes. What makes them look beautiful? They know how to put themselves together for an *impression* that drowns out a clinical analysis of their features or clothes. They've practiced, experimented on their faces and bodies, they've learned the beauty tricks—and they wear themselves as if they are legends.

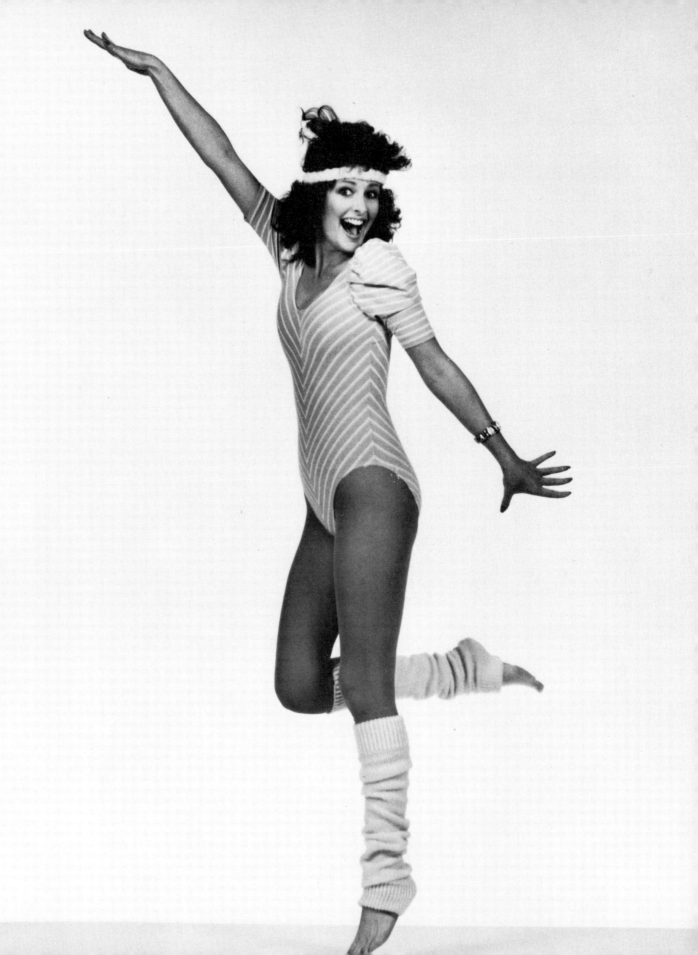

Chapter 3

LOOKING SLEEK WITH STYLE

The Attitude Diet and Exercise Plan

I COULD never make a life's work out of beauty.

Perhaps that sounds strange coming from someone who earns her living in front of the camera, but I'm convinced that there are so many deliciously sinful things about great food and great laziness that I could never banish them forever from my life. That's why I really believe that a woman with a size-eight figure, gotten from almost religious zeal of food deprivation and fanatic exercise, can never really look happily, magnificently beautiful—no matter how thin and firm she is. There is something more to life than deprivation. Thin thighs in thirty days can make you extremely cranky.

But I do believe in fitness and slenderness, joyfully and energetically obtained. It's possible to devise a diet and fitness style that takes your *humanity* into consideration.

Oh, I used to go on killer diets when my weight ballooned and I would starve myself to sickness to get back down. I would lead a Spartan life, develop punishing exercise routines, and, sure, I'd lose weight. I'd also be bored silly, not fit to live with, and very unhappy. There had to be a better way. I found it.

Two new ways of looking at food and exercise changed my life. First, the Golden Door, a wonderful fitness spa in Escondido, California, made me do some serious thinking about how to incorporate exercise and sane eating into my everyday life style—rather than go on repeated, frantic, perfectionist diets. Second, I gave myself permission to fail once in a while in this saneness. Permission to be human without hating my weakness.

To begin with, I'm very Italian. That means basically I'd rather be stirring noodles than be seen with the "beautiful people." I may have good bones in my face and a flair for life from my heritage, but it also means I have large hips and an unlimited belief in pasta power. My favorite room in the house is my kitchen. It has a huge, restaurant-style stove, a see-through refrigerator, and shelves and shelves of every variety of macaroni, spaghetti and linguine you can imagine. Neatly stacked, naturally. As a result, although I love fashion and style and svelteness, I've never had the typical model's body and I never will. It's not lean and rangy—it's rounded. I've settled for the fact that I'm not a willow reed—and what's more, my body changes as I get older. Yet I feel good, I know I look good, and I attribute it to a philosophy that has everything to do with liking and respecting oneself. In the end, all success is due to one thing: attitude. If you have a positive attitude toward yourself, you will have a positive attitude toward all of your life—and you will have a positive effect on others also. That's the secret of beauty. I can't promise that if you have a healthy and positive attitude you'll have a body like Christie Brinkley (I should live so long), or your boyfriend will come back, or your job won't be so confining, or you'll find your Prince Charming. I *can* promise you that *without* the proper attitude, very little will seem wonderful.

Having a positive attitude can move mountains. I am in the process of finding that out myself, right now, in an intensely personal way. "It's easy for someone to be positive when life is handed to her on a silver platter" was a refrain I'd often heard from my friends. Well, it was true: My life did seem to be charmed. I had a fabulous marriage, healthy children, a handsome husband, and money. If life was filled with valleys and peaks, mine was surely heavily loaded with the latter. I used to say to John that we were so lucky, God was going to zap us good one day—just to get our attention. I only prayed it wouldn't be one of the children. And then, sure enough, we got zapped—with a major zap. My charmed life and I were suddenly catapulted into a nightmare. My husband was arrested on a cocaine conspiracy charge that brought international headlines, false accusations, lies, and tormented children—my children. We weren't talking peaks and valleys anymore. It had become valleys and pits. It had become the real world.

Suddenly we weren't the golden couple. Friends disappeared. I'd been at the zenith of my profession for twenty years, but all the good looks, the goodwill I'd engendered, and all the money in the world couldn't explain the sudden loss of bookings. If ever I needed to fiercely maintain a positive attitude, it was now.

And it's working. Already the offers for covers are beginning to come in again. My life's work is currently picking up the pieces, forging ahead in every way—and, in the midst of "the troubles," keeping fit.

Back to attitude. I know that diet alone won't do it. I must be reasonable and know that I'm human and have human needs. Sure I have to watch what I eat, but I must also keep moving because diet without movement produces zilch. And, knowing myself and how important a strong attitude is with my own personal success, I must not allow myself to feel terribly deprived in my eating habits. I have a passion for excesses that comes upon me every once in a while and I accept that propensity for an occasional binge as natural. We've just lived through an era where looking good meant feeling lousy. The designers looked askance if you had a curve. Anorexic bodies and starved faces were the last word in beauty. I lost a sweet and dear friend, Karen Carpenter, to anorexia, the disease that came when she tried to fit everyone else's image of beauty.

Well, chunky's not exactly in, but we seem to have come, finally, to a more moderate approach. Exercise is a way of life and not a punishment for gluttony. Eating and staying reasonably, not cruelly, thin is a matter of moderation. Let me explain it to you another way. I'm a mood person. I have to be in the mood to do things right; otherwise, a halfhearted attempt always results in wishy-washy results. I have to be in the mood to shop, make love, or do my best work. I am, however, *always* in the mood to eat. I eat when I'm happy, sad, hungry, or not hungry. I have a major problem with food because I am a true foodaholic. Instead of having a binge with drink or drugs, I eat. I love food. I love to shop for it, prepare it, present it, watch other people eat it, and eat it myself. Underneath this high-fashion model is a potentially enormous, fat person. I've been suppressing her all my life. I have great respect for heavy women who can handle it securely, but *I* feel better mentally and physically when I'm thinner. It helps me retain that positive attitude I've spoken of. I carry myself taller, my clothes feel better, even my sex life is better. I'll be honest: It's always a great relief to me when I don't have to worry about covering my behind with a king-sized pillow when I leave the room after making love. It's always a relief to me when I don't have to worry about John grabbing thick mounds of flesh—how embarrassing! I hate having two wardrobes—one for pig-out periods and one for thin periods. But I've learned something about myself: I've learned that I must come to terms with dealing with a food obsession I will be fighting the rest of my life. It won't go away. So, I've changed my attitude about food itself—and dieting.

What follows, then, is the eating regimen I've found to be workable and humanizing—as opposed to self-defeating and depriving. It actually has four parts to it.

1. THE FERRARE PIG-OUT PLAN. This is the occasional binge I allow myself that keeps me from feeling deprived; that is, I never say "I will never eat Reese's peanut butter cups again."

2. THE ATTITUDE DIET. This is basically a conscious eating plan of having (more or less) about 900 to 1,200 calories a day in an eating pattern I take week by week. That is, I never say, "Today I'm starting a diet that will last until I lose ten pounds." How can one plan a serious weight-loss program *and stick to it* when every day brings a different set of circumstances? That's why almost all diet plans eventually fail—they don't allow for the *humanity* of a person's day-to-day life. An unexpected dinner party can wreak havoc on a strict diet; just the aroma of a culinary feast sends my head spinning so the best of intentions is forgotten when I show up for the dinner party . . . which gives you a good idea of my willpower. If I set limited goals (week by week) for myself, I don't feel as if I've failed when I break that diet if I just have to. After the "lapse," I go right on with the week's plan. Nothing is forever, and diets that are planned to last for longer than a week at a time *seem* like forever. This week-by-week dieting (or attitude dieting) doesn't have any set things to eat or any strict calorie limitations. I *try* to keep between 900 and 1,200 calories a day, but I don't despair if I go over that. I'll discuss this more fully in a moment, but for now, let's say that the attitude diet relies on *awareness*—being conscious of what you put in your mouth.

3. THE GOLDEN DOOR MAINTENANCE PLAN. When my Attitude Diet is going along pretty smoothly, I give it an extra zap by going on a special liquid diet one day out of every week. The Golden Door spa created it just for me, but anyone can adapt it to her own needs.

4. THE EMERGENCY DIET. Every now and then these first three parts of my eating life style have to be suspended for a true emergency diet. I save this drastic remedy (it's not really so drastic at all, you'll see) for when I *have* to get into a special dress or I know an occasion is coming up when I must lose four or five pounds in a week. If you opt for my emergency diet, you have to know that the results are not permanent. No one can permanently lose weight without changing one's attitude toward eating which means being consistent. The pounds you lose in a one-week marathon are temporary losses. Still, if you are in good health, and you check out the diet with your own doctor first, I earnestly believe that the emergency diet's a fabulous crutch to fall back on. You shouldn't do it too often because it's basically a liquid (although it's nutritionally pretty sound) regimen and one which is not *meant* to be standard fare.

Let me start telling you how I keep fit from the negative side of my fitness plan—*The Ferrare Pig-out Plan.* I know it sounds sinful and gluttonous and disgusting. I also know it's part of me—Cristina—my style, my vulnerability, my own way. In a funny way, it's as important to my life as my good-girl diet and exercise routines. What I'm about to tell you is fattening, teeth rotting and embarrassing—but curiously refreshing as the Schweppes man would say.

The Ferrare Pig-out Plan

About once every two or three months, you see, I get this urge to stuff my mouth, not with nutrition, but with junk food. I can always tell when it's coming. It'll never be on one of those nights when a nice green salad will satiate. It'll usually fall on a Sunday. I'll finish everything on my plate. Then, I'll eat what John and Zachary and Kathryn leave on *their* plates. Then I'll mosey into the kitchen and finish what's left in the pan. I can be up to my *nose* in food and I'll just keep shoveling it in because it's so good. Then comes the trouble. Once I start, I can't stop. I'm still *hungry*, you see, or so I think. I go into the kitchen and get some soft white bread from the freezer—the kind I never allow anyone to eat because of its nutritional deficiencies. It's only for my binges. This white-bread type of thing is forbidden to my children because of my nutrition consciousness. Yet I dig it out of the fridge, making myself a huge sandwich with gobs of mayonnaise, lettuce, tomato, bologna, salami, and I'm almost ashamed to tell you what comes next. I usually shove a few potato chips into that repulsive sandwich. The result is a huge, glutinous mess that I know in advance will stick to the roof of my mouth—let alone what it will do to my intestines.

I'm not finished yet. I wish I were, but I'm not. Confession is good for the soul. I get a *very big* bag of M & M's—not the measly little thirty-cent bag, but the giant Halloween trick-or-treat number. I pad up the back stairs of my apartment so no one, not even one of the kids, will see me, draw a warm, delicious Vitabath bubble bath, lock the door, get in the tub, and *glop down the whole bag.*

How's that for bad?

It gets more embarrassing to tell, but I vowed I'd be honest in this book. Last month I was in California visiting my parents. My father brought home a huge bag of Reese's peanut butter cups a friend had given him. Pack rat that I am, I hid them in a place where only I could find them. Every day I ate six or seven . . . and hid while I did it. When I disposed of the telltale wrappers, I shoved them way down at the bottom of the garbage bag so no one would notice them. When I left, I realized I'd eaten about forty-five peanut butter cups in a week's time. Oh, God—how mortifying!

It gets even worse. Sometimes when I'm home and I tell myself that because I'm feeling a little down, it's okay to eat, I'll sneak down to the pantry and get a plate of Häagen-Dazs ice cream (coffee, naturally), go to the trouble of toasting some coconut to sprinkle on top, put nuts on top of *that*, and chocolate syrup on top of *that* and glom the whole thing down while in the tub. Why I go to the tub to commit these sins, I don't know, except maybe that I subconsciously feel I have to cleanse myself afterward.

Have you ever sneaked into the kitchen at eleven at night to eat a croissant spread with cream cheese and fabulous homemade jelly? I have. The funny thing about it is that I don't *believe* in eating all that gunk! I am intellectually and morally outraged at myself when I put that stuff into my body. But it's that fat woman inside of me that's asserting herself every now and then—and I accept her, even if she's not my favorite part of me. So please understand that this book is written by someone who *understands* the struggle; high-fashion model and actress, yes; but very vulnerable woman also. Those lean and gaunt California beauties who can eat a dozen Mallomars without gaining an ounce have no right to lecture about how to keep thin. It's just too darn easy for them. On the other hand, if I tell you that a certain kind of eating pattern works—you'd better believe it! If I can do it, anyone can.

Naturally after one of the binges I've just described, I feel absolutely horrible. I have a miserable headache from the chocolate, my stomach aches, and I feel more guilt than *anyone* deserves. I hate myself.

So now you know the worst. Let me tell you the best.

For the next two or three months, following a binge, I *make* myself remember what I felt like. *After* the terrible sandwich. *After* the peanut butter cups. Although I can remember the good part of allowing myself a binge (and that *is* oddly satisfying), I also remember the fat, the headaches, the nausea, the fullness. It's enough to keep me very careful for a while. Careful enough to embark on what I call my Attitude Diet.

The Attitude Diet

It begins with a psychological lever. I actually *visualize* a thin, gorgeous me —the me that smiles on the magazine covers. I know she exists, as well as I know that the self-indulgent me exists. The trick is to concentrate on that slim me for a while. I remember, *very hard*, that No One Is Making Me Eat the Bad Stuff. That I *like* the salads and the good stuff. That a plain grilled fish in a restaurant or an endive-and-tomato salad with a little fresh lemon squeezed on it instead of heavy dressing is really out of this world. I leave jars of marinated cucumbers with fresh parsley and lemon wedges in the fridge—just ready for grabbing. I have appetizing bowls of fresh fruit sitting in my fridge—and raw carrot sticks and celery chunks in a bowl of iced water to keep them fresh and available and appetizing. I keep the picture of the slim and strong and pretty Cristina in my mind. And I begin a way of eating that doesn't depend on measuring food or denying myself— but which inevitably helps me to drop the pounds. It's a system that relies on *conscious eating.*

I call it conscious eating because it requires thought—not grabbing for anything that fits in the mouth. I *plan* a day's meals. I go for variety in foods because I know that boring foods can sabotage good intentions on a diet. I imagine myself eating, thinking, and moving like a thin person. I am not doomed by defeatist thoughts; I know that during these days of conscious eating if I munch on a Mallomar, I don't *have* to finish off the whole box of Mallomars. One cookie is not the end of the conscious eating days. I also consciously try to eat less of everything, even though I never deny myself a meal. Quick ways to lose weight, violent diets, don't ever work as well as eating a little of everything. You don't have to clean your plate. Honestly. And here's a tip: Cutting down on fats and increasing complex carbohydrates is the food lover's way to control weight. That means fewer proteins—less meat, less cream and milk and more grains, fruits, vegetables—even pasta, in moderation—minus the thick butter and sauce. It's funny —the first few days of my Attitude Diet are always a drag and a *little* bit painful. But once you start to see a physical change in your body, it gets actually exciting. You feel leaner, *harder*, sexier. You get to the point where you look forward to the conscious, thoughtful food decisions. It's a challenge.

Starting the day with conscious eating, I'll usually breakfast on some fresh fruit—papaya, melon, mango, oranges—whatever's in season, topped with cottage cheese and bran—and wash it down with some rosehip or herbal tea. For lunch if I feel like having a gloppy hamburger to keep my positive attitude, I'll have it—cheese, bun, and all—but for dinner I'll compensate with a small salad and a piece of broiled fish. What's the big deal? It's not so terrible, really. Want a piece of pizza? Have it—and get it out of your *craving*—just watch it at dinner. If I feel like having pasta in a restaurant, I'll have it, but maybe without the sauce and with just a bit of butter on it. It's not the linguine that will get you . . . it's the sauces you top it with.

I always think about what I put into my mouth, and unless I crave it, I order the healthiest, least fattening alternative. But if I *need* that hamburger? I eat it.

During this conscious eating, I weigh myself often—every time I go into my bathroom, actually. If I find that I've gained a pound or so instead of losing, I take smaller portions of everything, *but I still don't deprive myself of the things I love*. Doing that (and I went that route many times) would have me lose a few pounds of water weight fast and then, in despair and discouragement, gain everything quickly back. It is precisely that type of Spartan, martyr, deprivation dieting that inevitably causes 98 percent of all dieters to fail—and those are accurate statistics. My Attitude Diet includes the complex carbohydrates—nuts, fruits, vegetables, seeds, beans, and even starches! They provide more energy than protein-rich foods like eggs and meat. I'd rather eat a fettuccine-and-broccoli combination than a steak any day, and it's far better for me. Now, complex carbohydrates are very different from simple carbohydrates, which are usually just sugar sources. They provide important nutrients, fuel and fiber, or roughage, which helps the digestive system to function.

Why do I choose this kind of dieting instead of one of the myriad plans one reads about? Well, most extreme diets *do* work temporarily, but they can't work miracles and your own frustration and false expectations usually sabotage them anyway. It's far better, I believe, to eat a little of everything and balance your life with the understanding that weight changes as you do (your period, your aging, your emotional state), and if you're reasonable about your eating patterns, you're allowed to blissfully binge-gorge every now and then without disaster. I think that's the way to live a life of nutritional high style.

I might add here the personal game plan of Deborah Szekely who founded the Golden Door spa in California. She advises me (and her other guests) to stop, look, and listen before eating anything. Her theory is to *react* to food with intelligent consideration—rather than to mindlessly gobble it. I suppose that's where my conscious eating plan sprung from. After *stopping* the lunge for the doughnut, Deborah suggests that you *look* at it to determine how large the portion is and if the size relates to your size; does the food have life (as in a bowl of bright green grapes) or does it merely have sugar (as in Yankee Doodles). Most important, then, you must *listen* to the true messages of your body: Are you really hungry or do you just *feel* like nibbling; will you exercise today to work off the bagel; do you really *want* that melted cheese or will a salad make you feel better?

If you listen to your body's messages, says Deborah, it might tell you to take a swim instead of a sandwich. It might tell you that you're not even enjoying those potato chips you're mindlessly eating while watching TV.

Once I heard this saying: If God made it, eat it. If man made it, spit it out. Now, that might be overstating the case, but it's not a bad rule to follow. You can't get fat on salads. You *can't* get fat on fruits; even if they're sweet, because they're natural, they go through your system beautifully without leaving excess poundage. The food that grows in the ground, the vegetables, the greens—you're safe with them! It's the things that man makes: the pastries, the breads, the Milky Ways—those are the culprits! That also goes for most processed foods and most foods with additives, like bacon. Think pure, think natural, when you're on the Attitude Diet, as much as possible. But don't flay yourself raw if you dip into the potato chips every once in a while. Just make sure you really *want those chips*. Never waste the eating of a fattening thing if you don't really *need* it: save it for the Needy Times.

GREAT TIP: When I'm invited to a party, it almost inevitably sabotages my conscious eating. However, I've found a handy way to curb myself without putting a damper on my party attitude: When at a buffet, I use my dinner plate as a liner and my salad plate as the one on which the food is piled. I allow myself to take as much as I can fit onto that salad plate—I even pile it up artfully—*but no more.* You'd be surprised how much less you manage to eat when you cut down on the size of the plate.

Okay: Along with the Attitude Diet comes the Golden Door Maintenance Plan.

The Golden Door Maintenance Plan

It's never a pain, but a pleasure. It's so *good*, and it is a perfect once-a-week addition to my Attitude Diet. Once every week, I eschew most solid food and I prepare liquids that are comprised of solids, blended beautifully.

In the Early Morning: Grapefruit juice and decaffeinated coffee that I brew (not scoop from a jar). It smells like real coffee and sets me up for the day—I *need* that good A.M. coffee.

About 10:00: Time for another small glass of grapefruit juice or unfiltered apple juice. This glass keeps me going till lunch, which I'm eagerly anticipating. It also keeps my blood sugar up.

Lunchtime: In my blender, I put a mixture of sautéed (in sesame-seed oil) onions and four or five steamed carrots, celery stalks, or other vegetables I find in the fridge. I throw in eight ounces of low-fat cream cheese, defatted chicken stock which I always keep available in a plastic container in the freezer compartment, and my favorite seasonings: chives, curry powder, or an all-vegetable product. Then I purée the whole thing for a few minutes until smooth, pour it into a large soup mug, and I have a lunch that tastes like a thick, rich, cream soup. It satisfies my hunger and my urge for bulk. It's slimming and filling and fools the taste buds into thinking they're experiencing something sinfully fattening.

Afternoon Snack: (And sometimes, evening snack). This is the best concoction in the world. I throw whatever fruit there is in the house in the blender—bananas, melons, peaches, pineapple (either a combination or just one). I add a cup of nonsweetened apple juice and some crushed ice (this is very important—it gives thickness and a truly delicious consistency). When I blend the whole thing together, the result is the fruitiest, thickest, sweetest shake that tastes exactly like an ice-cream concoction but is not a millionth as fattening and a lot healthier besides.

Dinner: This meal is essentially the same as lunch, but instead of chicken stock, I use, for variation, some clear, defatted beef stock I keep frozen in individual serving containers for the same purpose. I'll also vary the vegetables, for a change of taste, but still throw in a bit of that low-fat cream cheese for the creaminess and thickness it provides. Spice it up with fresh chives, parsley or basil, a squeeze of fresh lemon and some pepper. Sometimes I heat the blend—sometimes, I have it cold. Whatever way it goes down, it is simply delicious and fulfilling. Somehow the combination of the liquid and the solid blended together is much more thick and filling than if I'd just had a bit of broth, a few vegetables and a drop of cream cheese, separately and in their solid state.

I think that if I did this more than weekly, I might tire of the richness, but once a week helps me maintain my weight without a feeling of deprivation. This liquid maintenance diet is so good and healthful that I often make double amounts for my family, who love it as much as I do.

The Emergency Diet

No matter how intelligent you are about your eating, no matter how you plan your diet in a reasonable way, every now and then comes the special affair, the interview, the date for which you absolutely want to look your very best. It means dropping four or five pounds in a week so you can fit into that new, dynamite dress in your closet. You *can* do it. Now, the Emergency Diet is just that—a one-week plan that is meant for sporadic and not regular eating patterns. It's kind of extreme (although not nutritionally unsound), and you wouldn't want to make it a life plan. Still, if you're in good health to begin with, and your doctor gives you the go-ahead, try this one-week regimen for instant results.

TIP: Don't think you're fighting your good sense with an occasional Emergency Diet. Even if you inherently disapprove of crash dieting (I do), think of it this way: Sure, sensible, daily conscious eating is the way to go. But sometimes you haven't been as sensible as you should be. Despite all your sense, you've gained eight pounds and you've just *got* to wear that dress next week. That's the real world. What to do? It's the Emergency Diet for you. *That's* the real world.

TIP: It's a very good idea to take vitamin supplements along with the diet, for energy and to replace any vitamins you might miss in your foods.

TIP: The more extra weight you have on your body, the faster it will come off in the Emergency Diet. If you are just about five or six pounds over your optimum weight, you may lose only about three or four pounds in a week. If you are ten or more pounds over your optimum weight, you'll probably lose up to six pounds in a week.

TIP: If your doctor agrees, you can continue this diet for an extra week, but don't make it a way of life; there simply are not enough solid foods in it to provide enough energy.

GROUND RULES

1. Drink as much water as you possibly can (at least six to eight glasses a day), but plan your drinking around where you're going to be. If you're out on the street without a bathroom in sight, soon after drinking a couple of eight-ounce glasses of water, you're going to be sorry you're living.

2. Try to eat or drink (the prescribed items on this diet) every two or three hours; that keeps you feeling reasonably full and it also keeps your blood sugar up.

BEGIN YOUR DAY A DISGUSTING WAY

Sorry, but you have to do it. During this diet, you eat very little solid food and you need something that will move what you do eat through and out of your system. I learned this from the Golden Door spa and it works wondrously. Daily, fill an eight-ounce glass with warm water (goes down easier than cold) and sprinkle two tablespoons of loose bran into it. Mix the water and the bran with a spoon and then *drink it down fast*. It tastes like sawdust and I hate it, but it "brushes your colon" as they say at the spa, which is just as important as brushing your teeth. It clears the system of toxins and the liquid foods you'll be eating and it's great for your skin tone as well. I try to do this almost every morning, not just when I'm on the Emergency Diet. I don't believe in artificial laxatives, and this is wonderful for elimination the natural way. Be careful that you drink your six to eight glasses of water daily, especially when you have the bran drink, because if there is not enough liquid flowing through your system, the bran can work in the opposite direction and clog you up.

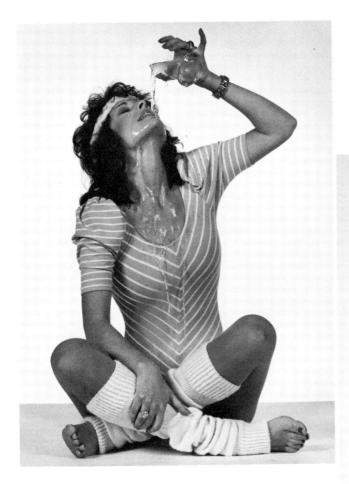

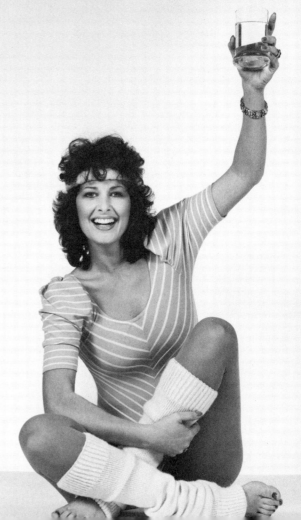

THE FIRST THREE DAYS

Breakfast: Even though these first three days will be a mostly liquid diet, I always eat breakfast so I feel as if there is some *substance* in my body. I enjoy a couple of eggs (you can cook them any way you wish, but limit yourself to one pat of butter), poached with a small slice of Monterey Jack cheese melted over them. If you hate eggs, substitute a bowl of fresh fruit and a couple of tablespoons of plain yogurt. One slice of whole-grain or bran toast and a four-ounce glass of fresh orange or grapefruit juice tops it off. I love good coffee, but I find the caffeine troublesome so I buy decaffeinated coffee beans, have them freshly ground, and the aroma of the brewing decaffeinated morning coffee fools me into thinking it's the real thing. I never deprive myself of a bit of cream either. The only thing I do without is sugar, which is really dreadful for you. Although I basically am not in favor of artificial sweeteners, I compromise and use just a tiny bit of an envelope of Sweet 'n Low (a whole envelope lasts me almost a week—that's how potent it is). I never use honey or anything like that because, although it's "natural," it has plenty of sugar and a whole lot of calories.

11:00: A four-ounce glass of any juice you like. If you put the juice in a blender with some ice, you get a concoction that's thick and frosty and infinitely more satisfying than just plain juice.

1:00—Lunch: Broccoli soup (or carrot curry soup or celery soup or any vegetable-combo soup) zapped up with your favorite spices (*not* salt). Following is a recipe for carrot curry soup. See the Golden Door Maintenance Plan (lunch-time) for another recipe. Use your imagination for other vegetable-soup possibilities.

CARROT CURRY SOUP

> 1 onion, peeled and chopped
> 1 clove garlic, crushed
>   Enough sesame-seed oil to coat bottom of pan (very little)
> ¼ teaspoon sage
>   Freshly ground pepper to taste
> ¼ teaspoon oregano
>   About 1 teaspoon crushed red bell pepper
> 1½ cups chopped raw carrots
> 2 cups (or more) defatted chicken broth
> 1 4-ounce package low-fat cream cheese
>   Curry powder to taste
>   Fresh parsley and chives to taste

Sauté onion with garlic in sesame-seed oil; add sage, freshly ground pepper, oregano, and crushed red bell pepper to sautéed onion. Add chopped raw carrots to mixture and briefly sauté again. Add two cups of defatted chicken broth to the vegetable-spice mixture. NOTE: If you have no broth, water will do, but it won't taste as good. Cook on low flame until vegetables are tender. Put into blender (not food processor) and purée. Add the low-fat cream cheese (half a cup of whole milk can be substituted) and about a tablespoon of curry powder (if you like the curry less "hot," use less) and blend further. Heat—but do not boil. Add fresh parsley and chives.

On a hot day, you can chill this outrageously delicious concoction and have a cold curry soup.

Now comes the important part: Serve yourself prettily. Put the soup in a lovely bowl or cup, sit down at a table and eat it lovingly. If you make a *presentation* out of everything you eat, you get twice the pleasure from it. What's more, you tend to eat more slowly, always more satisfying in a diet. Just glopping down this meal does it an injustice and, psychologically, you feel cheated of lunch.

With your soup, you can have some iced tea or lemonade, which you've conveniently prepared in advance and chilled in the fridge. Make the lemonade with fresh lemons and water and sprinkle in a bit of Sweet 'n Low when you're ready to drink it. *Never* buy a prepared lemonade, which is loaded with sugar. I use an herb tea instead of regular tea because regular tea has as much caffeine as a cup of regular coffee.

4:00—Afternoon Snack:
   A YOGURT SMOOTHIE. Take a half carton of plain yogurt. Put ½ cup *fresh* fruit in it (strawberries, raspberries, pineapple, banana—whatever you like). Add a four-ounce glass of unfiltered apple juice (which has natural sugar in it—not the added kind) or any unsweetened liquid you like. Blend it in the blender for an extraordinarily delicious treat.
   I can barely finish a yogurt smoothie and I'll often put what's left in the fridge to be enjoyed later in the evening.

6:00—Dinner: A soup again. Make something different from lunch and enjoy it with a hot or cold beverage.

8:00—Evening Snack: A four-ounce glass of juice. If you're really hungry, you can add a couple of celery or carrot sticks or a *tiny* piece of cheese, but be careful, because these add up in calories.
   And that's the first three days!

ON THE FOURTH DAY, and then afterward for the next three days, start *slowly* incorporating a little food back into your system. Do it gradually so as not to shock it. Have, perhaps, a large garden salad with a little lemon sprinkled on for dressing for lunch instead of the soup.

ON THE FIFTH DAY, treat yourself to a small, four-ounce veal patty for dinner. You can even melt a bit of cheese on the patty for taste. Eat some fresh steamed broccoli, fresh fruit, slowly and in small portions. Try to keep to 900 to 1,000 calories a day.

NOTE: You *cannot* shrink your stomach (despite the popular myth), but you can fool your brain into thinking you're satiated on a lot less than you usually eat.

And that's your Emergency Diet week. During the first couple of days, you'll probably lose the most weight—that's water loss. Don't be discouraged if you don't lose as much as you'd like; it didn't take a week to put all that extra weight on, and it may take more than a week to lose it all. Still, you should be very satisfied with the immediate amount you manage to drop, and happily, you should be able to get into the dress for the big occasion.

A WORD ABOUT EXERCISING DURING THIS WEEK

During the first few days, because of the reduced solid food, you will probably feel a bit weak and not up to your usual exercise routine. Keep moving though, even if you have to cut it down a bit. You can exercise while you're *sitting* in front of the TV or reading a book (see the chapter on exercise for leg raises with a three-pound weight and other sedentary-type exercises). As you eat more solid food, beef up the exercise.

IT WON'T KILL YOU

You may find that you're slightly "headachy" during the first few days. Don't worry about it. My own doctor says that that's a symptom of the toxins leaving the body via the "bran drink" and other liquids.

AND ONE FINAL IDEA ABOUT DIETING, IN GENERAL. AND I'M *NOT* KIDDING:

I've always thought that a great way to impel oneself to diet is to eat a meal or so *stark naked*. If you have trouble finding the willpower to cut down on junk foods, eat dinner in the buff for a few days. You'll be surprised how encouraged *not to gorge* you'll be.

Whenever you're on *any* kind of diet, certain rules prevail.

Bloat Battle Strategies

BEST BETS

• Always have a light appetizer ready before dinner (tomato juice, crudités, and so on) to cut down on hunger at the table.

• Order *plain:* pasta without cheese sauce, salad without oil dressing, steamed instead of creamed vegetables, popcorn without salt and butter at the movies, baked potatoes with plain yogurt and chives instead of sour cream. . . . Soon you get into a *rhythm* of eating plain (even though you eat almost everything), and that makes the difference. You even get to appreciate foods in their purest forms—a delight, long lost in a world of sauces and salts.

• Reevaluate your thinking about food. Food is not an enemy. It's not an all-or-nothing situation, a *never*-cross-your-mouth-with-fattening-foods situation. Thin behavior relies on a moderate, satisfying approach—eat everything, but only a *little* of everything.

• Drink camomile tea; it's a natural diuretic. So are watercress and asparagus.

• Alcohol on hot days seems to promote bloat—so say my two martini-drinking friends. I don't drink so I don't have this particular problem.

• Cut down on the stuff that goes *on* food. Salt is a killer, makes your body swell from water retention. Try using lemon instead of salt, toasted sesame seeds instead of sauce, dill weed instead of mayonnaise. Sauté with wine or unsalted soy sauce instead of oil or butter.

• Keep staples in the house for on-the-run snacks and meals (you tend to eat oatmeal cookies because they're *there*): foods like tuna packed in water, fresh fruit, low-fat yogurt, and low-fat cottage cheese, are fast, grabbable and relatively unfattening. See? Are you getting into the habit of attitude dieting? Measuring or weighing foods is not natural. Besides, you *know* what's too much to eat. Twelve chicken thighs are too many.

• Do away with excesses. A bagel, for example, can be sliced by your grocer into six bagel thins. One is very satisfying when you crave a filler with a cup of coffee, and it takes three days to eat a whole bagel that way.

continued on next page

WORST BETS

• When you want to look your thinnest, avoid the foods that produce gas, which puffs up your belly. Among these foods are cabbage, notorious beans, cauliflower, broccoli, and carbonated drinks.

• Why would anyone want to drink Coke (five teaspoons of sugar) when she can drink Tab with lemon (no sugar)? However, don't overload on diet drinks. I always feel that if I can't pronounce what's on the label, I should drink very little of it.

• Don't shop when you're starving. That's how the Hershey's Big Blocks get stowed away in the house. Only shop after you're *full*.

• Emotional crises don't get better when you're eating éclairs. The lover doesn't come back, the boss doesn't relent about the no-raise decree, and the cold doesn't get cured when you stuff your face. Better buy some new makeup for a lift.

• Peanuts and potato chips at bars, hors d'oeuvres at parties will do you in, every time. They ought to be outlawed.

REASONABLE BETS

• There are one or two other points to be made about feeling fit. I'm a great believer in vitamin supplements. Every day I take four tablets: a multivitamin, a stress vitamin (either B_6 or B_{12}), an iron supplement, and a vitamin C. The kids all get multivitamins, as well. I often take a calcium supplement in pill form rather than in milk or cream form because milk is very mucous-forming in adults.

• I sleep about seven hours a day, rarely longer, get a physical checkup twice yearly, and brush my teeth three or four times a day (I've only had one cavity in my whole life!).

Finally,

The Dieting Social Strategy

I've learned that there is nothing in this world more aggravating than a person who doesn't shut up about her dieting. If you want to lose friends fast, tell your hostess's other guests why they shouldn't eat the mousse. Keep your hunger pangs to yourself. And don't be so virtuous that you're a pain in the neck. Eat *something.* Push the food around on your plate. Don't count calories out loud or on your handy little pocket calculator.

If You Don't Use It, You Lose It!

This is the section of the book that deals with exercise. Let me make a general statement first: I *hate* those virtuous beauty-book authors who complacently tell me to exercise an hour a day. Now, come on, give me a *break*. Who has *time* to put in a whole hour a day? I figure twenty minutes a day of planned exercise is terrific—and anything else I can squeeze in, while I'm watching television or reading, is gravy. Sometimes I *think* I'm tired or nervous, but a brisk walk does me a lot more good than a tranquilizer, a nap, or a drink would—which is why I don't drink or take pills (and naps are a great, but rare, luxury).

I think it's important to set aside a time of day when you'll put in those twenty minutes, *every* day. For me, it's about 4:30 in the afternoon, when I'm usually home from modeling assignments. In the early morning I tend to want to get on with the business of the day and I'm too excited and motivated to stop for exercise. At 4:30, I'm winding down my day and exercise gives me a lift for the evening hours. Of course you must decide what the best time is for you, and the important thing is to stick to that time. If I'm in a good mood, I'll put in longer than the twenty minutes, and that happens a couple of times a week. But I find that if I exercise when I'm sitting in front of a TV, when I'm lying in bed reading, when I'm talking on the phone—those minutes add up and before I know it, I've put in close to an hour almost every day. A friend of mine once told me she'd been dieting, she figured, for about twenty years, and had gained eight pounds from it all. That's because she didn't exercise along with the dieting. I know as surely as I know that my name is Cristina that you *have to* exercise that body to keep in shape. Scientists change their minds every twenty minutes about what drugs are good for you, and what kind of counseling best helps your psyche, and even what *kinds* of exercise are the most fruitful—but there's one thing they never change their minds about, and that is the fact that some kind of exercise is essential to everyone. Every bit of movement, every time you walk up a flight of stairs instead of taking an elevator, every single time you do leg raises with weights as you watch television (or even during the commercial) helps to keep your body slim and fit. I don't think that most overweight is a result of overeating anyway; I think it's a result of undermoving. Labor-saving devices, and a generally sedentary way of life are doing us in—no kidding. Sometimes it's inviting to sit lashed to a chair, I know. But I try to keep *something* moving, almost all the time I'm sitting, even if I just stretch my leg out eight or nine times in a row. You have to earn the right to enjoy total slothfulness—by putting in your movement time every day. Think of exercise as a job that *must* be done.

I've told you about my favorite room—my elegant, big, and useful kitchen. I have another favorite room. It's my exercise room. Bare floors, exercise mats, a record player for inspiration, and pictures of my children, paintings that I've lovingly created are all that are in it. It represents a positive, happy life style. When I visit my exercise room, I think I realize an amazing sense of self. I am saying: "This is a time that's uniquely mine; giving myself a half hour in this room daily not only shapes my body but allows me to tap energy I didn't know existed, and, thus, physically renew myself."

I didn't always know this or understand it. You're reading the words of a former *total* sloth who never earned the blessings of a fine body and health, but who, instead, was born with good genes. I never once stopped to worry about: Would it last? Would *I* last? I was making top money, lauded every day for my beauty and body, and I accepted this good fortune without questioning it.

And then, the biggest miracle of my life happened. After trying hard for a long time, I became pregnant with my daughter, Kathryn. It was a difficult Cesarean birth, there were many hormonal changes in my body taking place, and I was blown up out of proportion. Instead of being admired by men for my beauty, all of a sudden I had a matronly image. You know how men are when you're pregnant—they *respect* you so. Well, it continued after the pregnancy. There I was, supermodel, actress, dream girl—turned blimpo. One hundred and fifty pounds of blimpo. Instead of the admiration, I'd get pats on the head from men. My husband was extremely supportive—the "I'll-always-love-you-even-though-you're-fat" kind of support—but I hated myself. And what's more, I didn't feel as energetic, strong, or healthy as I did before. I knew I had to get moving.

But first, I tried the excuses. . . .

- What, *me* exercise? I'm so busy, I hardly have time to breathe.
- I think I'm coming down with a cold. Also, my period. I'll start tomorrow.
- First, I'll lose ten pounds—then my exercise program will be meaningful.
- It's raining out. It's terribly hot. I look lousy in a jogging suit. I don't *have* a jogging suit. Zachary needs help with his homework. I read where you can hurt your back, get a prolapsed uterus, sprain your ankle—oh, it was something—with exercise.

But even I wasn't convinced.

So I made a few uncoordinated and very fitful starts. I'd go to a spa that plunged me into exhausting exercise that they said would burn up fat—but not only did the brief plunge into movement *not* burn up fat, I knew the Olympian calisthenics were never going to be part of my life style. I'd write out hefty checks for health club memberships that I never took advantage of because they required going someplace special, and I was always too busy or too lazy to get myself to the special place. Writing the check to the health club did not notably decrease the size of my can or even increase my wrist's muscle tone. In California, I sat around the pool a lot, but that only helped minimally.

I got chunkier and I had serious doubts that I'd continue to be an inspiration to people who still thought of me as a glamorous cover girl.

And then came a moment of truth. I realized I had the power to change. I'd worked very hard to get where I was, and if I only put the same energy into keeping fit, I'd succeed. I knew one thing for sure—punishing and sporadic starts and stops wouldn't do it. I'd have to find a routine that fit my life—that didn't bore me—that I could be consistent with. And I did.

One of the biggest secrets of my exercise routine is that it changes. I don't do the same thing every day, because the sameness of the routine would soon make me discard it. But generally speaking, this is it—with variations every now and then to relieve monotony.

Exercises for the Happy and Fit Woman

First of all, it always helps if you can grab a kid to exercise with you—or a friend, or a husband. My children and I often go through a morning stretch routine together. It provides inspiration and companionship. If I miss a morning, I feel stressful and anxious, and I'm jumpy at work and with the kids. The morning stretch exercises are not the true exercises, but they get the sleepiness out of my system. I warm up for the day this way for about fifteen minutes.

THE MORNING STRETCHES

First, I stretch up—high, high, to the ceiling—then stretch to one side, then to the other. Then, bending from the waist, I touch my hands to the floor and

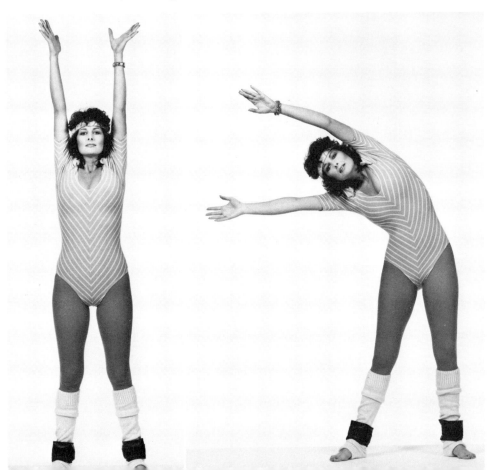

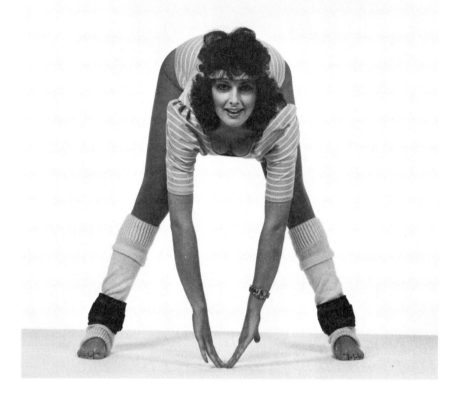

stretch (never bounce on a stretch; you can hurt or tear a muscle if you're not warmed up first). I do this series about fifteen times and it tones my muscles without creating hard muscle masses. The kids and I always listen to music as we're stretch-exercising—either a classical music selection or some contemporary Melissa Manchester–type of thing. Next, in a changing pattern, I usually sit down with my legs stretched out in front of me and bend into them, touching my

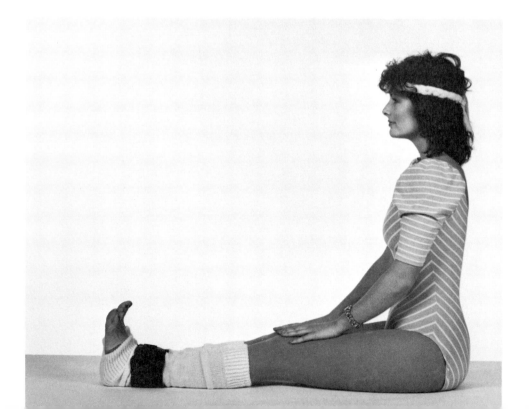

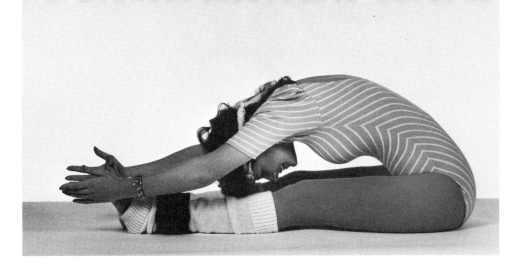

toes and beyond the air (also about fifteen times). Then, standing up, I stretch my arms overhead and clasp my hands together, then stretch to one side, then the other—about twenty times to each side. I stick to the bends and stretches in the morning, but Kathryn usually does her own thing which includes the most amazing variations of jumping, stretching, and pulling to the music. That usually does it for the morning.

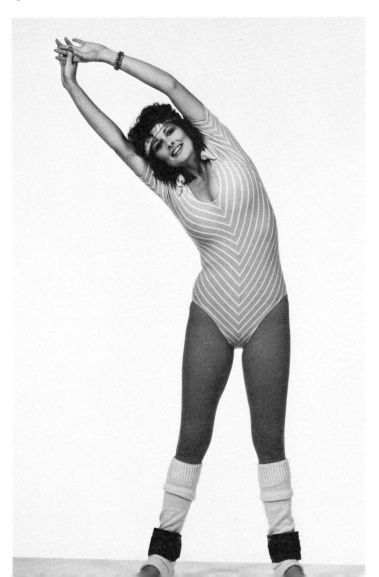

In the afternoon, usually at about 4:30, I do my serious spot exercises and aerobic dancing. After a brief warm-up stretch (just a few of the morning stretches), they usually include the following exercises (and others I may pick up along the way).

Start slowly and work up to the maximum!

NOTE: Many of these exercises call for the use of weights. Only use the weights two or three times a week. On the other days, do the exercises without the weights.

THE REAR END WHITTLE

I put a three-pound weight on my ankle (any sporting goods store has them), get down on my hands and knees, and lift the weighted leg to the side and up—about twenty times. Transfer the weight and do twenty lifts with the other leg. (Try to keep your torso as straight and as still as you can.)

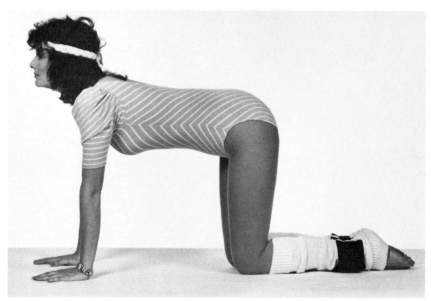

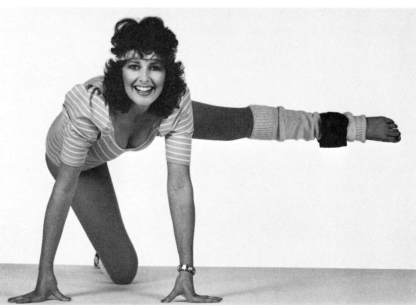

THE THIGH WHITTLE

Lie on one side with your hands on the floor in front of you for balance. It helps to flex the knee of the leg on the floor for better leverage. Lift the weighted leg up as high as possible, and then lower it. Do this ten times then change sides and repeat with the other leg. This exercise works the inner thigh muscles beautifully and trims off fat. The buttocks get a workout also.

If you do the same exercise but only lift the leg halfway up, the outer thigh gets the most concentration. If you lie on your side and lift the weighted leg straight up backward, the buttocks "saddle bags" and the lower back muscles are worked very well.

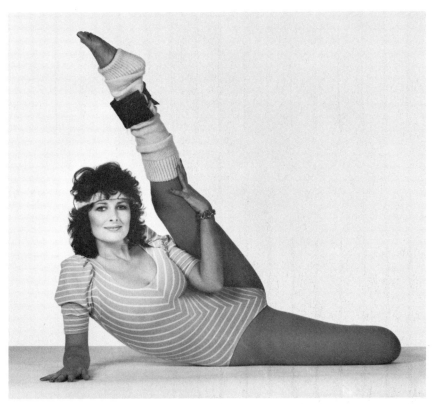

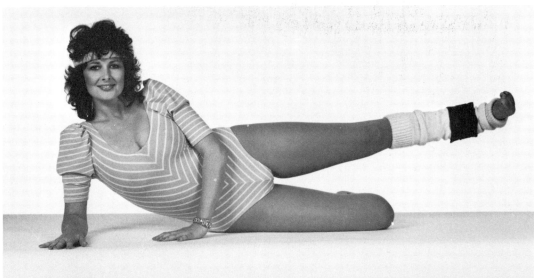

97

THE ELBOW-KNEE TWIST

This is great for flattening the abdomen and strengthening the back and upper body. Lie on your back on the floor, clasping your hands beneath your head and bending your knees. With your hands still clasped, lift your upper body and knees simultaneously and try to touch your right elbow to your left knee. Alternate, touching your left elbow to your right knee—twenty times to each side.

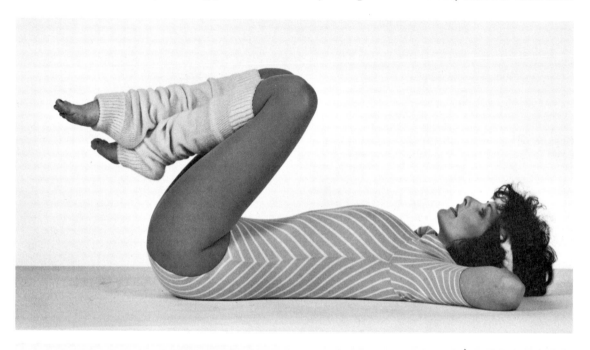

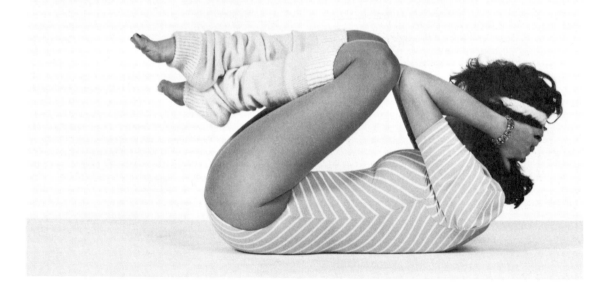

Swimming is, of course, a wonderful all-around exercise that trims down every part of you: the thighs, the upper arms—everything. I love to swim for its all-over body conditioning and for the skeletal muscle build-up. But sometimes a pool's not so handy. In that case, I'll do an on-land stroke, which tightens and strengthens the backs of my shoulders and also relieves neck, shoulder, and back tensions.

THE LAND SWIM

This tones the upper arms. Hold a two-pound weight in each hand (a book will do). Stretch your arms high overhead, then pull them back in a wide half circle to shoulder level, as if you were getting ready to do a dead man's float on your back. Continue the circle, keeping the elbows straight, and bring the arms straight back as far as possible, then down, then straight out in front, as if you were preparing to dive. Return to the overhead position. Do the land swim twenty times in a smooth and continuous motion.

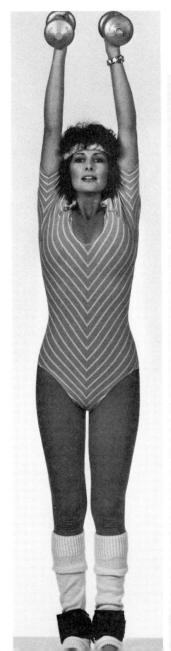
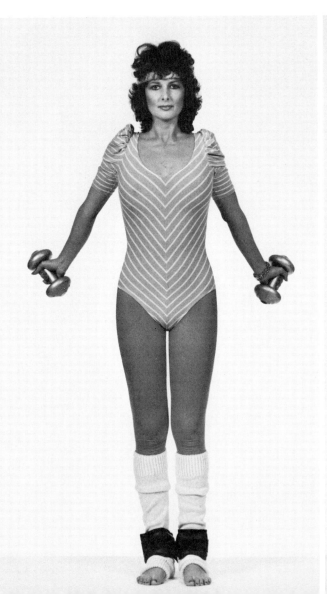
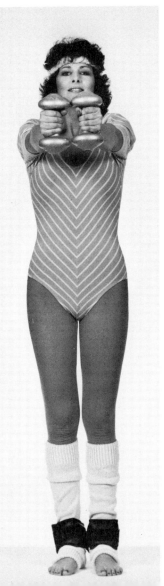

THE SCISSORS

This exercise flattens the tummy and whittles the thighs. Lie on your back on the floor, bend your knees and place your hands under your buttocks. This supports and cushions the back muscles. Lift and spread your legs in a wide V.

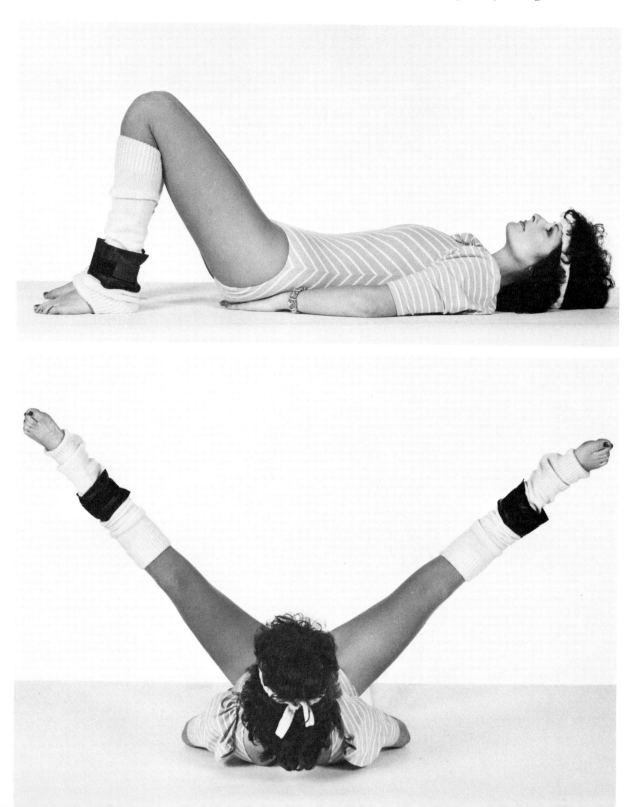

Keeping your lower back pressed to the floor, lift your head and shoulders, point your toes, and, keeping your legs straight, "scissor" them, crossing at the knees. Then open them as wide as you can in another V. Start with fifteen scissors and build up to twenty-five. You can do a scissors kick while you're sitting or talking on the phone with a buddy. Don't waste a minute!

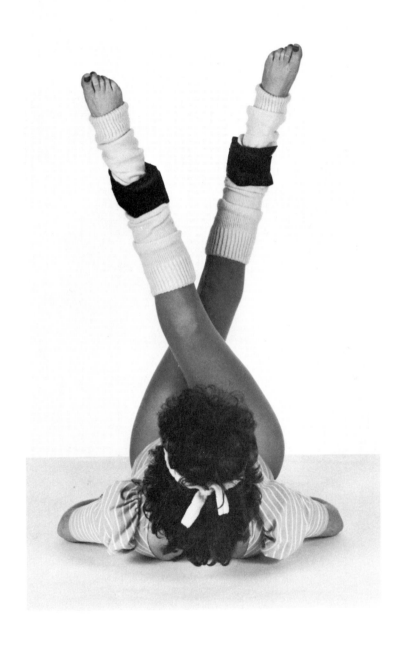

THE TUB TIGHTENER

You're tightening your tummy and back muscles—not the tub. Lie on your back in your bathtub, resting on your elbows. Keep one knee bent and that foot on the floor. *Slowly*, lift the other leg as high as possible and then lower it. Do ten times for each leg.

NOTE: If you're not in the mood for a bath, this exercise can, of course, be done on the floor.

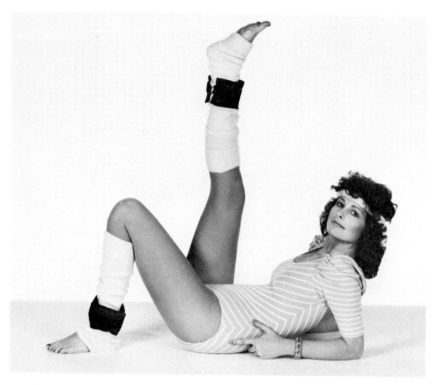

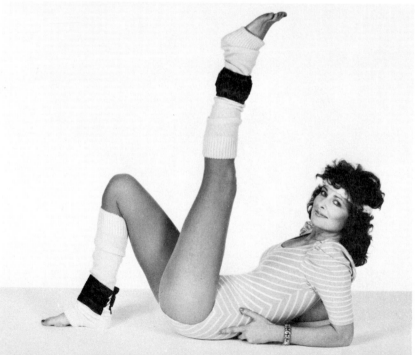

THE THREE-IN-ONE

This is a Waist Whittler, Inner-Thigh Trimmer, and Outer Thigh Tightener.

Sit on floor with your legs wide out in a V, feet flexed, and your hands close in flat on the floor in front of you. Extend your arms between your legs, keeping your elbows slightly bent. Without bouncing or jerking, try to touch your forehead to the floor and hold that position for ten to thirty seconds. (It will be *very* difficult to get your head all the way down at first, but build up over a few weeks' time by bending the head forward as far as it will go until you can actually touch the floor.) Straighten up to starting position and then bend at the waist to the right, stretching your left arm and head toward your right foot. Sit up straight again and then stretch to the left, extending your right arm and head toward your left foot. Repeat the sequence eight to ten times at first and gradually build up to twenty.

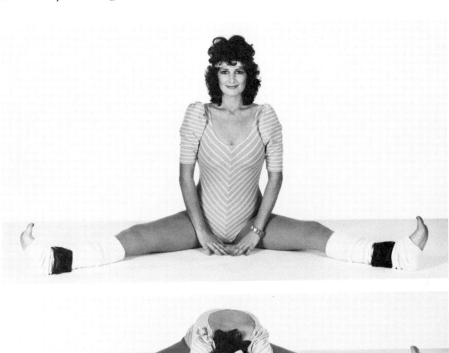

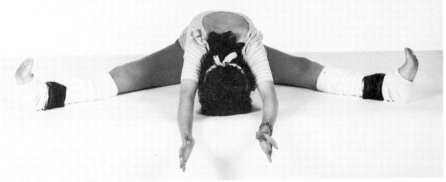

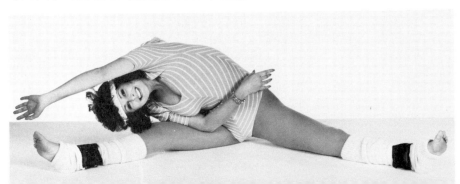

103

THE BUN WARMER

Here is a rear end killer!

Lie on your back flat on the floor, with your hands out at your sides. Bend your knees and keep your feet flat on the floor. Suck in your stomach muscles. Now squeeze those pelvic muscles tight and lift your pelvis for a slow count of twelve. Relax and lower body to the floor. Repeat twelve times. With pelvis lifted, separate and then close knees ten times—great for inner thighs.

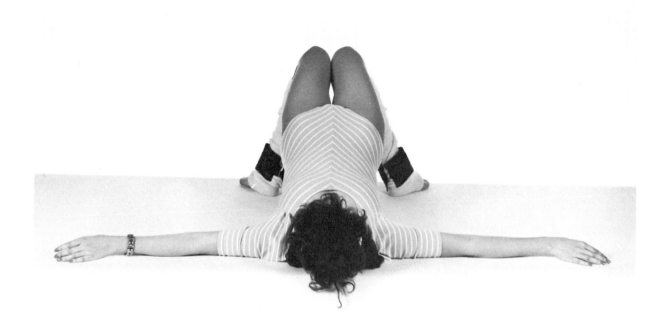

THE FLAB-AWAY

This is an upper-arm tightener.

Hold a two-pound weight or a book in your left hand. Sit Indian-fashion on the floor with your legs crossed at the ankles. Raise your left hand, holding the weight overhead, and grasp your elbow with your right hand. *Slowly* lower the weighted hand in back of your head, bending your elbow to do so. The weight will pull down your hand to your lower neck. Raise weight; repeat the sequence ten times, and then repeat with the weight in right hand.

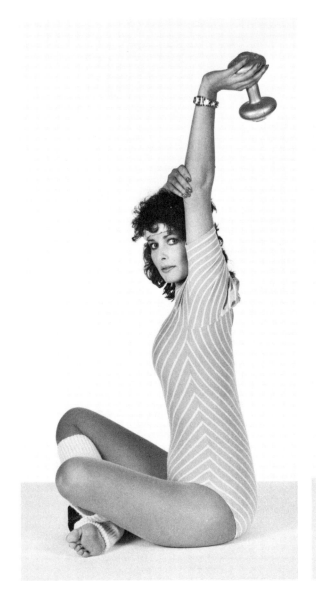
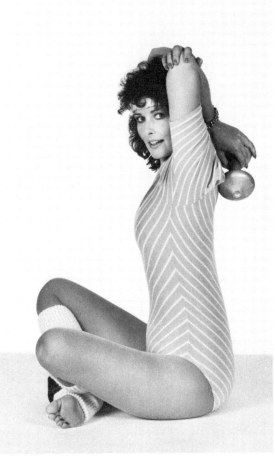

THE AEROBIC SHAPE-UP

Here we have an all-around circulation booster. After a series of spot exercises, I always do a session of aerobic movement. You must do aerobic exercise without stops and starts. It does wonders for the whole cardiovascular system, gets your lungs working at their peak, and moves that blood through your body. The thing to know about aerobic movement is that you have to do it for at least eight to ten minutes straight to get any benefit from it. You do *not*, contrary to thought, have to work up a sweat to get the fat-burning benefits, either, but you do have to keep it going for a while. Kathryn and I love the new aerobic dance records; Jane Fonda puts out a good workout record that includes a whole routine. Richard Simmons has one, and even Miss Piggy has an aerobic exercise workout routine album. Sometimes I just dance fast, or jog to any fast music with a good beat.

Exercising, for me, is not confined to an exercise room or a special time. I rarely sit in one place without moving a part of my body. I do arm circles and deep knee bends while chatting on the phone. Moving is a way of life for me, a habit, a part of me as necessary as breathing. Fantastic promises of weight loss through imaginative diets are just that—promises, not the truth. Dieting can't work unless you move. Time spent in the bathtub without feet flexing, time spent without tightening and loosening my abdominal muscles when I'm waiting for a table at a restaurant, time spent without leg raises while I'm waiting for a photographer to set up a shoot is lost time for me.

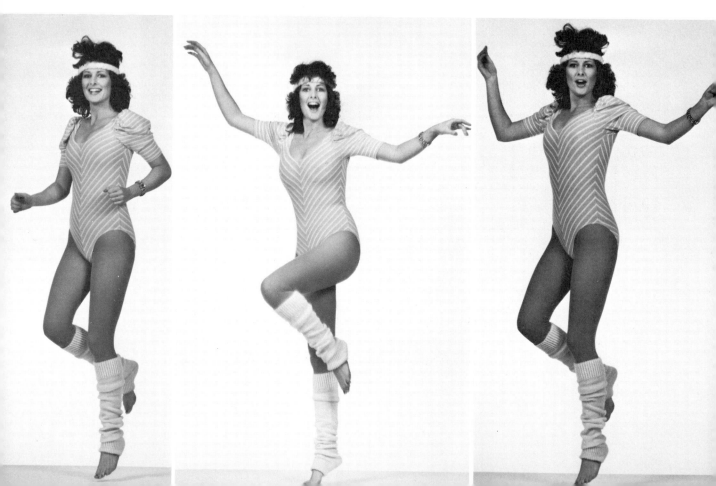

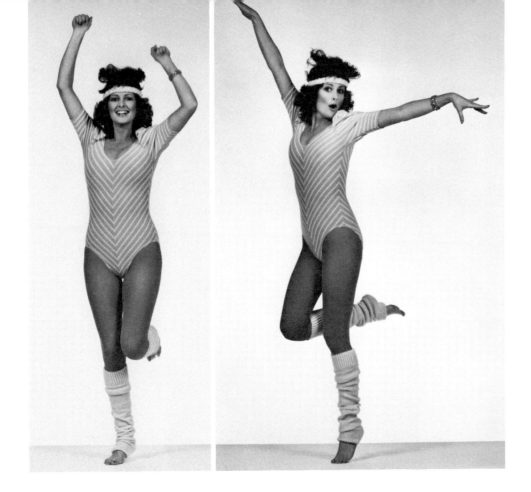

Things You Should Know About Exercising

1. Work up to the maximum. If the exercise calls for twenty stretches, start with as many as you can without straining and gradually increase the number every day.

2. Exercise slowly and correctly; don't rush through the routine. The idea is to lift those legs, stretch those arms gently and in continuous, slow motion. Jerky, fitful, swift stops and starts defeat the purpose of creating muscle tension and release. The only exception is that aerobic exercising has to be done faster and faster as you build up endurance. Everything else should look as if a slow motion camera had photographed an exerciser under water. Fluid, slow, continuous.

3. Keep breathing, inhale and exhale regularly; fight the tendency to hold your breath during an exercise.

4. Don't ever forget about your legs while exercising to improve physical fitness. The late famous cardiologist Dr. Paul Dudley White once said, "You'll never get fit just using your arms. Each leg is an auxiliary of the heart. Each leg is worth half a heart in maintaining maximum circulation during the activity" (which means, when you swim, *kick*).

Exercises You Can Do Without Ever Leaving "Magnum, P.I."— Keeping Fit While You Sit

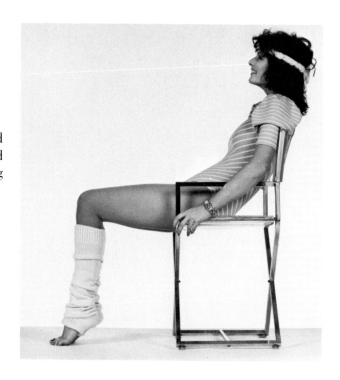

Sit in your TV-watching chair and slide your bottom slightly forward. Hold the chair for balance when not using your arms in an exercise.

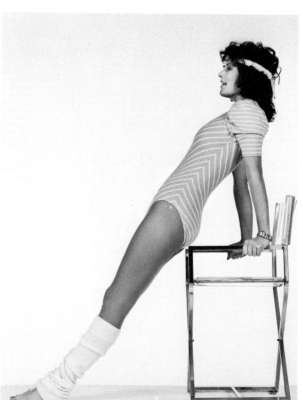

1. FOR FIRMING THE UPPER ARMS. Keeping your feet on the floor, grab the armrests with your hands and push down with your hands to lift your body off the seat and hold for about five seconds. Lower to the seat and repeat three times.

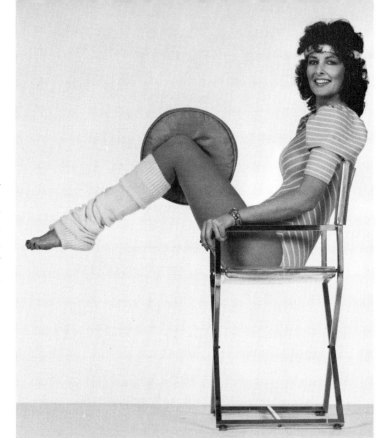

2. GREAT FOR THE ABDOMEN AND THIGHS. Sit back a little farther in the chair. Put a small pillow between your knees and lift it up as high as you can. Hold for six seconds. Keep your toes pointed and squeeze the cushion hard. Repeat three times.

3. GOOD FOR THIGHS AND CALVES. Sit deeper into the chair and bring your left knee up to your chest. Next, point your left foot up toward the ceiling and *stretch*. Do ten times, then repeat with right leg. Don't rush this one: It takes several weeks of practice to point that leg straight up!

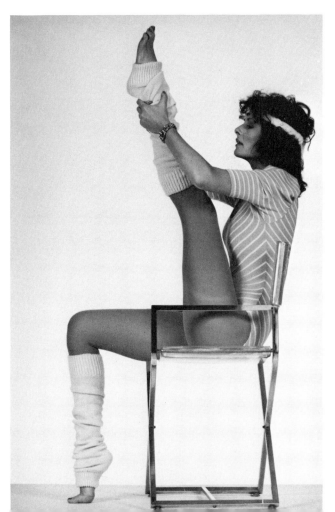

4. GREAT BACK STRENGTHENER. Squeeze your buttocks *hard* together and hold for five seconds each time. This exercise can also be done while lying in bed, waiting in lines, or standing on the bus or in elevators. Work up to twenty to twenty-five buttocks squeezes.

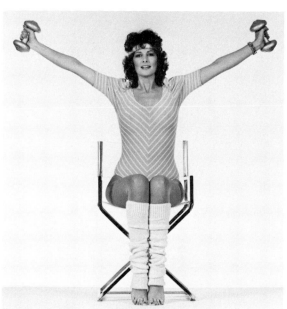

5. FIRMS UPPER ARMS. With a two-pound weight in each hand, stretch your arms to the sides and make ever-getting-larger-circles in the air. Do ten circles in a forward direction and ten in a backward direction.

6. TO FIRM UPPER ARMS AND STRENGTHEN BACK. Lift both legs off the floor and cross them at the ankles. Raise your arms (keeping elbows straight) widely above your head and bend your wrists so your hands point toward each other. *Slowly* bring your hands together until your fingers touch, and then extend your hands outward again. Repeat ten times.

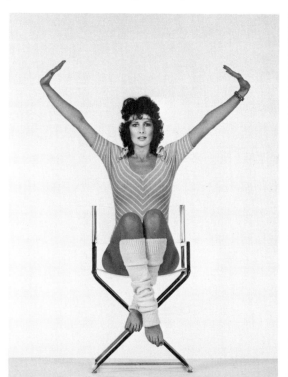

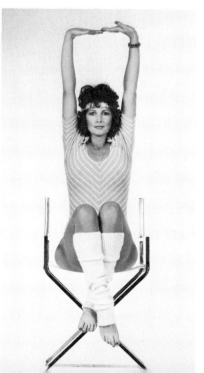

7. TO TONE INNER THIGH MUS-CLES AND STRENGTHEN LOWER BACK. Sit forward slightly in the chair, grasping a small pillow between the knees. This time point your toes downward and raise and lift the pillow continuously, barely touching the floor with your toes on each "down" movement. Repeat twelve times and build up to twenty-five.

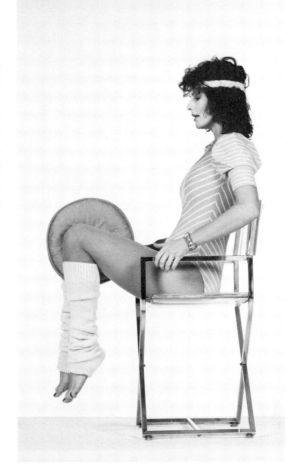

Exercises for Posture

The way you hold your head and shoulders when standing or walking is the difference between slouch and stride. There's no such thing as a sloucher model because if you put the most beautiful woman in the world in the most exquisite clothes on the runway, and she looks as if she has what we used to call "dress-maker's hump"—*forget* it. She won't do justice to the clothes, won't project glamour and health, won't be rehired. Posture means everything to style and grace. Let your mirror be a camera lens: Stand a good ways away and move toward it. How do you look? If you move like an orangutan, you need to work on your posture. We know from painting and sculpture that posture is often used by artists to depict an emotional state, a power message, or an image of beauty. The powerless, the sad, the depressed, and the unbeautiful are often crouching, shoulders rounded, on canvas or in stone sculpture. Learn a lesson from this and do exercises specifically geared to induce good posture. The following are adapted from suggestions of Dr. Joseph M. Lane, associate professor of orthopedic surgery at Cornell Medical School and chief of metabolic bone disease at the Hospital for Special Surgery in New York City. Go through each exercise, starting by doing the movement once and then working up to ten, twenty, or more repetitions, depending on your stamina.

1. Lie on your back with bent knees and your feet flat on the floor, clasping your hands beneath your head. Bring both knees toward your chest and hold for a count of five.

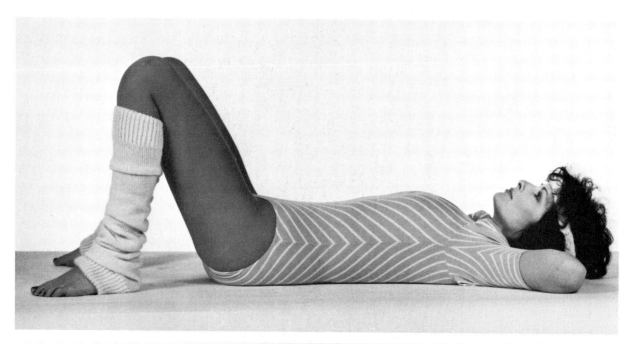

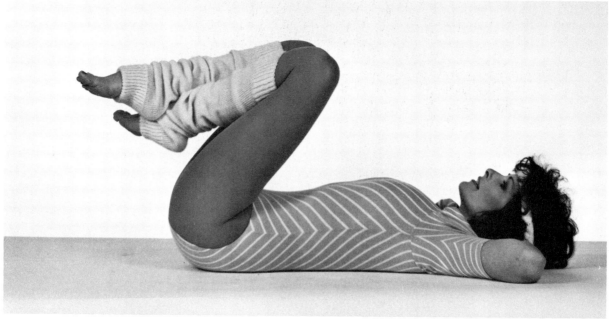

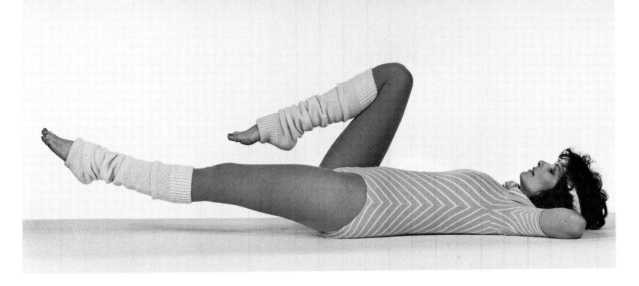

2. Start in same position as exercise #1. Lift your right leg—keeping your knee bent—and bring it toward your chest. Then extend your left leg straight out until the back of your knee is flat. Keep the extended leg a few inches above the floor. Hold for a count of five. Return both legs to the starting position and repeat with opposite legs.

3. Start in the same position as exercise #1. Flatten the small of the back against the floor by tightening the buttocks and stomach muscles. Hold for a count of five.

4. Lie on your back on the floor with one knee bent and that leg's foot flat on the floor. Raise the straight leg six to twelve inches off the floor and then lower it slowly. Repeat with the other leg.

5. Lying on your back with knees bent, feet flat on the floor, and your arms folded across your chest, bring your head and shoulders up toward your knees. Raise your head and shoulders only, not your whole torso. Hold for a count of three and lower slowly.

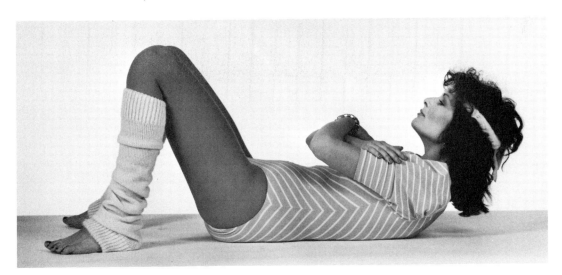

6. Lying on your back with your legs straight, knees together, and arms at sides, bring your head and shoulders up toward knees. Raise your head and shoulders only, not your whole torso. Hold for a count of three and lower your head slowly.

7. Start in the same position as exercise #1 but with your arms folded behind your head. Bring your knees to your chest and immediately return to the original position, but don't touch your feet to the floor. This is a continuous and smooth movement. Repeat.

8. Lie on your back with your legs straight, knees together, and hands palms down under buttocks. Raise both legs six to twelve inches off the floor. Hold for a count of three and lower slowly.

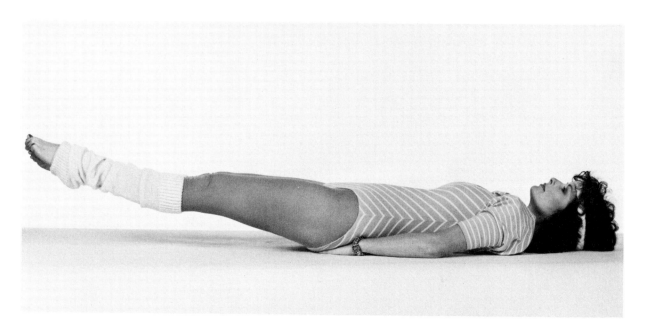

9. Lie on the floor with your knees bent, feet flat on the floor, your hands clasped behind your neck, and elbows pointing to ceiling. Stretch elbows slowly down to floor. Hold for a count of five and return to the starting position.

These exercises will help to strengthen your back as well as induce you to carry yourself straighter. They can be done while talking on the phone, watching television, or in bed.

Posture depends on the straightness of your spine, and even if you've always had miserable posture, you can resurrect that spine at any age—so don't give up hope. Stand against a wall, press your spine against it, and look into a mirror: Now try that without the wall. Keep a picture of that look in your mind when you walk stairs, down the block, and even when you sit. Another of my private practices for posture is this: I've hung a "chinning" bar in my closet, wall to wall. Every now and then I just hang from it (grasping tightly with my hands) and that stretches and elongates my muscles, relieves back tension, and helps me stand straight. The most stylish look in the world is simply eradicated when you schlump along! By the same token, physical grace can mask too many pounds or unattractive clothing.

Gracefully Getting Into and Out of a Car

Speaking of physical grace, here's a bonus tip for you that you probably won't read anywhere else. Where's the hardest place to maintain physical grace? Getting in and out of a car, of course! It simply defies most people's ingenuity. Forget one fluid movement: Even Greta Garbo couldn't get out of (or into) a Honda (or a Cadillac) in one fluid movement. But I know how to do it—getting in, go fanny first. If you should even attempt to do it foot first, your body will end up in a hopeless tangle—skirt riding up to your thigh. Stand with your back to the car door and sit down on the edge of the seat. Your feet are still planted on the sidewalk. It is helpful to lightly place the hand that's nearest to it on the dashboard, for balance. Then, with your weight on the outside foot, swing yourself and your inside foot around and into the car, following with that outside foot. You're in! Neatly and gracefully, I might add. To get out, swing both legs around and place your feet on the sidewalk (or street) so that while still sitting you're facing out. With the hand nearest the back of the seat resting on the seat, simply duck to clear the doorframe and stand. You're out! The look of grace is further established if you keep those shoulders straight instead of contorting them during the in-and-out-of-the-car motions. You can duck by inclining your head and shoulders in one fluid movement instead of hunching those shoulders inward.

For the Exercise-Really-Gives-Me-a-Pain Person—The Therapeutic Walk

There are always some of you out there who start out on an exercise program with the best of intentions—and who inevitably fail to be consistent. You get bored with the whole thing, deny that you have fourteen minutes a day to spare, and resist any *planned* time stubbornly. For these people, it is the height of self-delusion to keep making new resolutions and, just as quickly, to keep breaking them. In the end, one has to know one's own patterns and if you are not going to exercise *every day*, you might as well forget the self-promises. *Sometimes moving* means zilch. But all is not lost. There is always walking. It is perhaps the best exercise in the world and the most interesting because you have the world to look at as you walk. In order to get some cardiovascular benefit from a walk, you really have to bop along at a pretty rapid rate—none of your sauntering, window-shopping walking. But, to add variety, you can adapt a wardrobe of walks.

Try

- an *angry* walk—fast, hard steps and a serious arm swing;
- an *athlete's* walk—a long-stepped, bounding walk;
- an *ethereal* walk—kind of a float that doesn't let your full weight sink down on any step.

A combination of these makes walking more interesting, gets your muscles moving, your blood pumping. Plan to walk to work, to lunch, to at least one place every day if you simply will not exercise. It won't make you much thinner, probably, but it will make you healthier.

That, then, is my program. It works. If you combine conscious eating with daily exercising (making allowances for an occasional pig-out), you *will* look sleek, you *will* feel good. Starvation dieting and exhausting exercise don't have to be your style.

Me, Me, Me, Me, Me. Only Me.

And then there's one thing more to feeling fit. It's called Selfishness. I'm not talking about throwing-the-other-guy-out-of-the-raft kind of selfishness so you get to keep all the food and water. I'm talking about renewing your spirit, your psyche, kind of selfishness. It's a soul massage. Taking care of your own ego, your tautness of spirit, includes relieving anxiety and tension. I simply must be alone for a while to do this. My aloneness consists usually of an after-vacation (usually Christmas and Easter) flight to the Golden Door. It's self-indulgent, but it's necessary to recharge my batteries, think things out, be without the responsibilities of home and husband and children for a while. I love to just sit around, talk girl talk with my friends, do silly, stupid stuff. It helps me see my life and work in a different light. I always know when it's time to go because I start to pig out more than just occasionally. The last time it happened, I'd said to John, "Do I look fat to you?" "No," he answered tactfully. "Not fat. Just thick." Thick!! Oh, no. It was off to the Door. There I exercise, meditate, get glorious massages, hang out with girlfriends. But such a sybaritic experience is expensive and costs time as well as money. If you can't afford a trip away, a trip to your bedroom, *alone*, or to the bath, works almost as well. Also, there's nothing as rejuvenating as turning out the lights and lying down for a quick catnap that doesn't necessarily have to include actual sleep. It does require aloneness and total removal of kids, dog, and telephone. Sometimes I refresh myself in the bathtub. When I sit in my

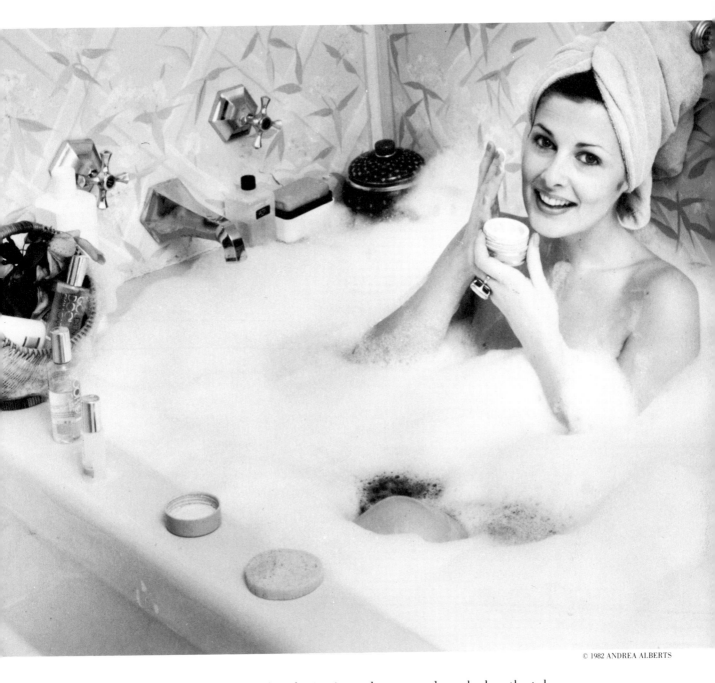

bubble-laden oasis with a glass of iced juice in my best crystal perched on the tub edge next to me, flowers (fresh, of course) on the windowsill and a good, meaty book in my hands, I somehow find my lost core. An hour of quietness, treating myself with respect and pampering, is worth a five-hundred-dollar course in Transcendental Meditation. I have trouble with mantras, if you must know the truth. I can't let my mind wander long enough to be successful with yoga. What I do very well is escape—for a week or an hour. It gives me a new lease on life.

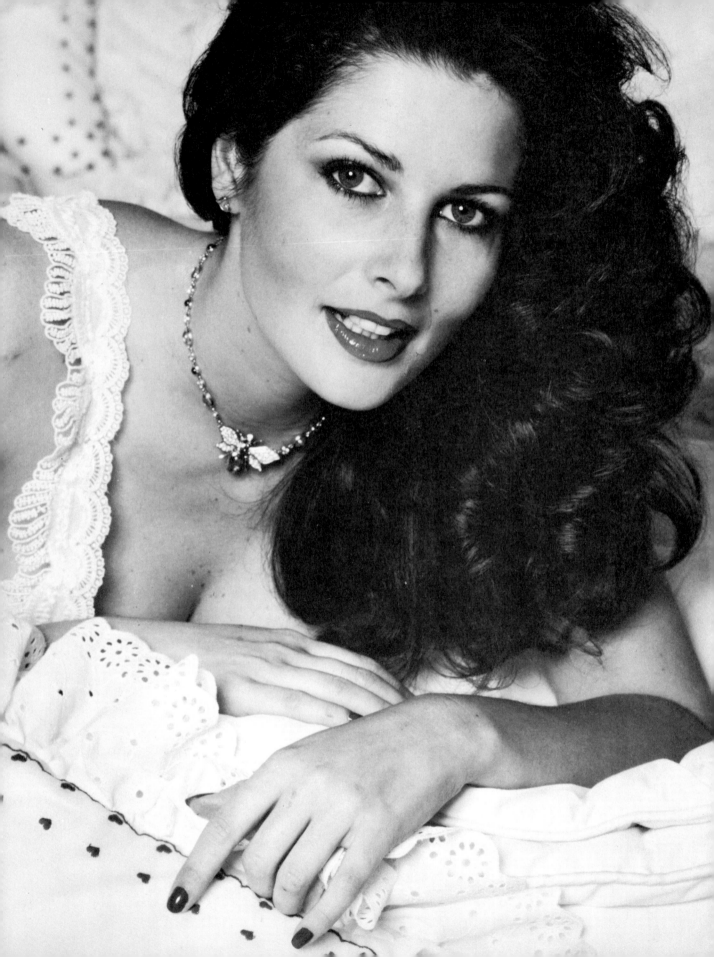

Chapter 4

HAIRSTYLE

Wonderful Hair

RECENTLY I went to an art exhibition that featured the poet Walt Whitman's original manuscripts, his pipes, his pen. It was all very interesting—until I got to the lock of white hair that was once growing on this bard's head—and then, it was *electrifying*. There's something about hair that personifies the essence of an individual. It's so personal, so alive, even though it's made up of dead cells. When I wake up on an "off" day, if my hair looks terrific—I look terrific. On the other hand, I can be primed to go, with a perfect makeup and a dress of the highest style, and if my hair looks crummy, nothing works.

Hair. You can bleach it, dye it, frizz it, color it, curl it, puff it, wave it, shave it—and it always comes back for more. It's so *durable*, when you think about it. In the newspapers the other day there was a story about some archaeologists who'd dug up an Egyptian eighteenth-dynasty mummy from about 1400 B.C. She was almost gone, naturally, except for leathery pads that were once her skin, shreds of linen that were once her ball gown—but, unbelievably, a mass of the most silky, voluptuous red hair remained. Every single other manufactured thing had turned to dust, every human feature was obliterated, but you could still see what a beauty she was from that hair that had lasted throughout centuries.

For myself, a new haircut or hair look gives me a lift. It's better than a tranquilizer and a lot less fattening than my beloved pasta. During a recent emotionally devastating time of my life, one of the first things I did was to go out and get a drastically different haircut. Up until then, my hair had been long, loose, kind of pre-Raphaelite. Now, for some reason, I wanted it severe, short, tighter. I really don't know why—I just *needed* the hair change for my psyche. The press, of course, had a field day. They said everything from "She had the haircut so she wouldn't be easily recognized in the street" to "She had the haircut to give her a Joan-of-Arc suffering look." Nothing could be further from the truth. That week I would have been recognized even if I wore a blond fright wig. More than anything, I wanted to hide my anguish—*not* proclaim martyrdom. Somehow, instinctively, I knew a haircut would soothe, would be more right at that time. It was. It provided a new look and a feeling which gave me a crazy kind of uncomplicated source of strength. Such is the nature of hair.

What is the nature of *your* hair? If you know your hair type, you know what kind of shampoo to buy, what to expect from a haircut, and how to best care for your hair. You can find out your hair type easily by asking yourself the following questions.

How to Find Your Hair Type

1. *Does your hair take a set quickly, then droop afterward? When it's humid out, does your har drop limply (or frizz up like a halo if it's naturally curly)? Is it stringy? Does it fly away easily and have plenty of static electricity?*

You have fine hair. It will do well with a conditioner that will "thicken" it by coating each individual hair. A body wave or permanent will give it substance. Stick with a blunt cut (all the same length) if your fine hair is straight, because a layered cut can make it look skinny and sparse. If it's curly, though, layering will give it plumpness and direction. Blow-dry it small section by small section instead of in larger sections. Fine hair looks best shorter; keeping it long encourages the weight of the hair to flatten it out.

2. *Does your hair hold a set wonderfully well—for even a couple of days? Does it do the same thing pretty much all the time, depending on how you cut and set it?*

You have medium-textured hair. You're in luck—it's the easiest to deal with. Cut is all important, so spend your money on finding a hairdresser who's famous for cut, rather than color or high style. Once your hair is cut (either layered or bluntly), you can experiment with almost any style. Electric rollers work very well; always use end papers to avoid split ends and excess drying.

3. *Does your hair have problems taking a curl even with electric rollers? Is it bushy, unmanageable, and wild-looking much of the time?*

You have coarse hair. Because it weighs more than fine hair, it can fall flat as well. But the weight of the hair can be a plus with the right hairstyle. A precision blunt cut will add lift, but if your hair is curly, it can stick out with layering and you can have too boxy a look; try a body perm—just on top—and get yourself a good natural-bristle brush. A cream rinse will give you control.

4. *Does your hair look greasy if you are not meticulous about a daily wash? Are you plagued by dandruff?*

Your hair is oily. The hair follicles secrete more than their share of oil and sebum, and scaliness, itchiness, and white flakes appear. Shampoo daily. Use a dandruff-controlling shampoo; they're the only shampoos that are really different from the others. Avoid hot, hot water and keep your blow dryer on low because heat stimulates oil glands.

5. *Is your hair supercharged with electricity, flyaway, dry to the touch, brittle?*

Your hair is (no surprise) dry. Treat it gently—use electric rollers only once or twice a week, tops. Pat it dry, never rub it vigorously. If your hair is dry, your skin is probably dry also, and a vaporizer or humidifier, which puts moisture in the air while you work and sleep, is a good bet. Avoid too many *things* done to your hair in the form of permanents, tinting, bleaching (never color and permanent your hair in the same day). Cut off split ends to avoid the split going farther along the hair shaft. An after-shampoo conditioner may temporarily put some substance into your hair, but it won't stop dry hair from splitting. The conditioners and creams are just bandages—not cures. Dry hair tends to look dull, because the hair, an extension of the skin, can also "peel" off in layers from sun, water, and chemical damage; as the cuticle is chipped away, the hair loses luster. Condition it and brush it gently to shine it up.

Tricks of the Modeling World

Every doctor knows the easiest way to stop the bleeding; every model knows the most direct route to the illusion of beauty. When your hair doesn't look great, nothing else does. Here are some tips and touts I've picked up from myriads of colleagues during the course of countless shootings on the

Cleaning,

Conditioning,

Combing,

Coloring,

Cutting of hair.

Cleaning

The longest you can go without a hairwash is two, *maybe* three, days. The minute it looks scruffy—wash it! Clean hair is a psychic energizer. Dirty hair weighs you down.

NATURAL SHAMPOOS

For light, dry hair: Steep some camomile tea in a cup of water for about twenty minutes. Beat an egg yolk into the tea and lather it through the hair. Rinse well.

For light, oily hair: Same as above, but use the egg white instead of the yolk. Substitute lemon juice for camomile tea.

For dark hair: Use the above recipes, but instead of camomile or lemon, which are natural bleaches, use sage or rosemary infusion with the egg; they tend to enrich dark color and make it more vibrant.

THE MODEL'S OIL-OUT EMERGENCY SPECIAL

Assume your hair is very oily, even though you've washed it just an hour ago. Assume, also, that the audition director has called—you've been scheduled to make a trial commercial before the morning's over. Try this: Dab some talc or baby powder on the roots of your hair and brush it through. Your hair is cleaner, dryer, fresher looking almost immediately!

FOR DANDRUFF

If you seem to be losing hair and gaining dandruff, don't worry; the loss of hair is pretty normal—most people lose up to one hundred hairs a day. Dandruff is not so acceptable. Try a shampoo that's formulated especially for dandruff (Head & Shoulders works well). Or see a dermatologist. Sometimes dry dandruff is caused by having a water-poor scalp. *Drink*, drink, drink to moisturize. Scalp massage smetimes beefs up blood circulation and that often helps.

Conditioning

For dry or brittle hair: Try a castor-oil conditioner made from two tablespoons of castor oil and one tablespoon of olive oil. Warm together (not too hot for fear of the old oil-boil torture), massage into your scalp, and then brush through the hair. Wrap your head with steaming (not *too* hot, again) terrycloth turbans for about twenty minutes. Keep changing them so they stay hot. The oil will penetrate your scalp and moisturize the hair. Shampoo very thoroughly after the treatment.

For normal hair: A coconut oil conditioner works wonders. Heat two tablespoons of coconut oil (get it in a health food store) with a beaten egg and a tablespoon of cider vinegar, and massage it into the scalp. Cover your head with a steaming turban for fifteen minutes. Shampoo and rinse.

For blond oily hair: Take a half cup of lemon juice, a beaten egg yolk, and a cup of water. Massage it into the scalp and hair, leave it on for five minutes, then rinse *very* well. You can finish up with a bit of lemon juice and water poured onto the hair and left there.

For brunette oily hair: Blend a handful of watercress with one cup of water in a blender or food processor. Boil the mixture for ten minutes, strain out the watercress, and cool. Apply to damp, clean hair, leave on for fifteen to twenty minutes, and rinse with cool water. The watercress plant is wonderful for leaving hair oil-free.

THE MODEL'S VITAMIN E SPECIAL—A DAMAGED-HAIR RESURREC-TION TIP: Many models I know whose hair has been damaged or made brittle by too much heat from rollers resort to a simple 400–international unit vitamin E capsule which they mix with a few tablespoons of soybean oil. They apply it to the damaged ends and comb it through all the hair. Then they put on a heat cap or sit under a dryer for about ten minutes, shampooing the whole mixture out afterward. Rinsing with cold water adds shine. The whole process seems to restore the hair almost instantly.

Coloring

What are . . .

TEMPORARY RINSES? They're semipermanent color treatments that shampoo in and last for about six shampoos (even though the manufacturers always say they last for a shorter period). If you've never colored your hair before, or if you just want to tint a little gray, this is for you. Temporary rinses don't lighten hair—they darken it. Always do a patch test before using a new product (try a small area first to see if you're allergic to the coloring or acid additions in the rinse).

PERMANENT DYES? They're not really permanent because they only last until the new hair grows in. They include henna, peroxide and/or other chemical substances and can lighten or darken. They don't wash out.

FROSTING, TINTING, HAIR PAINTING? These lighten or darken only strands of hair and give contrasts, highlights, and touches of color. They're attractive when the technique picks up the natural variations and tones of your own hair and worse than preposterous when you clunk a patch of blond color on a head of coal-black hair. You *must* consider skin tones when you're changing hair color. Golden tones in ash-blond hair are often stunning; henna-mahogany tones on wren-brown hair can be rich and lustrous; brunette flashes in Carol Channing hair are definitely not attractive. And take it from me, you must consider your own aptitudes before doing it yourself. If you're not by nature terribly handy with your hair, like me, let Marge (or Suga or Richard) do it. Amateur-looking color jobs on hair are really terrible. Aside from lemons and one or two other "natural" coloring agents, it doesn't make much sense to pour coffee, beets, onions, or food coloring on your head as I've heard some do. How can hair smelling of coffee be seductive?

HOME COLOR WASHES

Although only a professional should ever make serious color changes on your hair, here are a few home "brightener" techniques that are quite popular in the modeling world. You can give them a try just for fun.

For very blond hair: Blond colleagues of mine make a shampoo-bleach mix using half shampoo and half twenty-volume peroxide. They lather it into wet hair, let stand for five minutes, and then rinse and condition.

For light brown hair: An herbal potpourri of a tablespoon of rosemary, a tablespoon of nettle, three tablespoons of Aloe Vera gel and just a touch of peroxide, left on for ten minutes and then shampooed out, works nicely.

For very dark hair: Ordinarily I hate putting stuff like coffee on my hair (many beauty books recommend it to wake up the darkness), but a glass of grape juice mixed with shampoo and then shampooed and rinsed out after about ten minutes gives a lush smell and is a wonderful temporary color brightener.

QUESTION

How come my raven-black hair looked fantastic when I was nineteen, and looks tacky when I color it the exact color at forty-three? It *is* my natural color.

ANSWER. Natural is one thing at nineteen and quite another at forty-three. As you pile on the years, your skin loses some of its natural color—just as your hair does. The raven-black hair you wore at nineteen is not natural for you today. Somewhat lighter hair is more flattering as we age. By lighter, I don't necessarily mean blond. Blondes do *not* have more fun, even though they're easier to find in the dark.

Combing

- Broken combs can break your hair.
- So can teasing or back-combing.
- If your hair is thin, there's a trick that models use to make it seem twice as thick in bulk: Lean forward from the waist with your head bent down. Brush your hair from the neckline forward. Spray the undersides of the hair lightly with hair spray and stand up. Lightly brush (or even just finger-comb it) into place.
- Combing the hair today requires mostly a brush and a blow dryer; very few women sit still for the indignities of pin curls and rollers. You don't need five thousand attachments either; just a simple "gun" type dryer. A vent brush is wonderful because air is able to move through the brush and facilitate the drying process.
- *Keep away from hairDOs.* You know what I mean—Dorothy Hamill-dos, Lauren Bacall-dos, and so on. Hair*dos* always make you look like someone else. That's not what I mean by style. Instead, look into the mirror. Tousle your hair. Look at it from every angle. Be the best *you*, not the best *do*.

Curling

ELECTRIC ROLLERS

In a pinch, when you need fast curls, there's nothing like a set of electric rollers. The bigger the roller, the fuller and looser the curl, and the more time you leave it in your hair, the tighter the curl. Wait until the hair has cooled after removing the rollers before you comb it out.

HAIR CAN RESTRUCTURE YOUR FACE

For a Large Nose. A backward sweep of the hair, off the face, makes it look smaller. Try a ponytail or chignon.

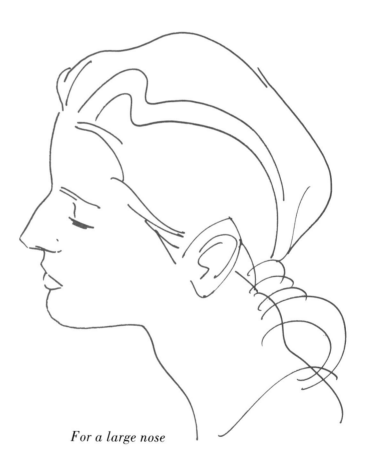

For a large nose

For a Very Small Face. Fuller, rounder hair is flattering—accomplished with a great, short haircut.

For a Low Forehead. A severe, straight-back-off-the-face hairstyle looks best.

For a High Forehead. Wisps of bangs or full bangs shorten the height.

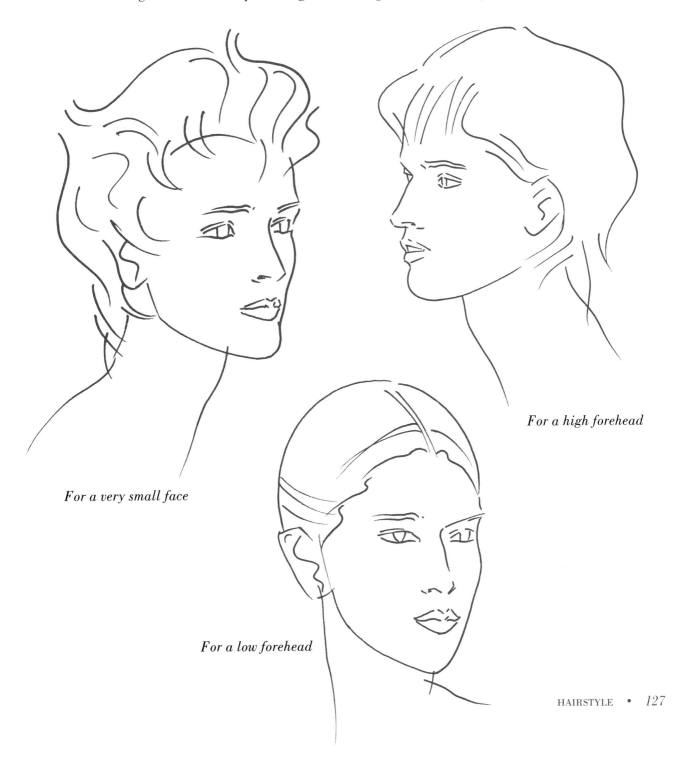

For a high forehead

For a very small face

For a low forehead

For a Round Face. Try a center part with hair falling across your forehead and cheeks, *gently*—not bouffant.

For a Jutting-out Jaw. Short hair curling onto the face below the cheekbone detracts from the prominent jaw.

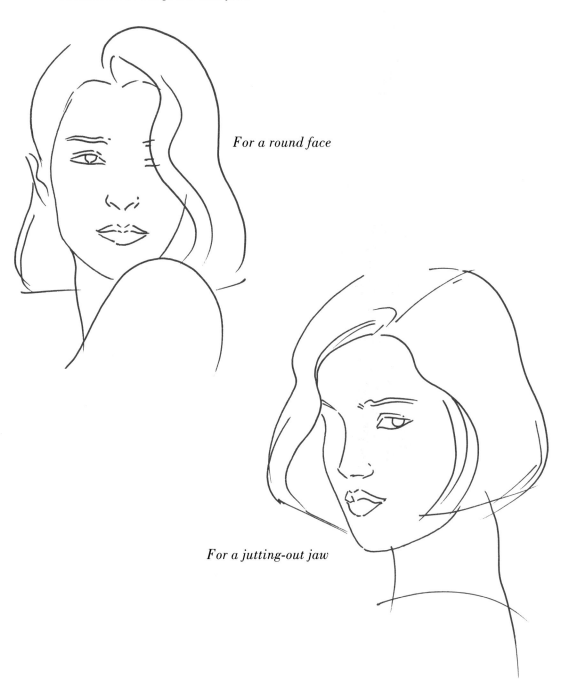

For a round face

For a jutting-out jaw

Cutting

The absolutely one essential thing you must get is a good, no, a *Great*, haircut. A great cut will allow you to shake your head while dancing and still have the hair return to a swingy, appealing shape. It's the difference between looking fine, even after you've been caught in a rainstorm, and looking like something the cat dragged in. It's the difference between being able to take a swim at the beach and having to sit, pristinely perfect, for fear your hair will get crazy. I hate to have the hair fall in my face (when it's long) and I hate to have to keep *fooling* with it during an evening out. Probably the clearest example of *un*-style is taking a comb out at a dinner table (or anywhere in public) to restore damage. Everyone hates to see that and I think men hate it most of all. A great haircut solves all of those problems. That's why it's worth it to pay a small ransom for a good haircut, travel a long distance or wait in a long line. Give up the new dress, the play, the book, the weekend vacation or lunch for a month to pay for a good haircut. Do *not* let your best friend hack at your hair unless your best friend is named Suga.

HOW TO CHOOSE A WONDERFUL HAIRDRESSER

First of all, before you make a drastic move with your hairstyle, do your homework and become familiar with the work of the hairdresser you plan to use. Never get a whole new look from someone who has never worked on your hair before and is not aware of its personality. Even a very skilled artist can give you a haircut that transforms you into Little Orphan Annie if he doesn't know of your hair's ringlet propensities. So have the hairdresser experiment during several preliminary appointments—shaping, guiding, blow-drying your hair—while you see if you like his or her touch before the day of the Big Cut. And, before making a big style change, look at your hair from every angle. If it's long, hold it short. Fool around with wigs at your local department store to see how you look in the hairstyle that looked so great on Brooke Shields in that movie.

HAIRDRESSER PLUSES AND MINUSES

• It's not important (a) how beautiful his salon is; (b) how expensive he is; (c) how much of a wit he is; (d) how friendly (or how quiet) he is; (e) how famous he is.

• The very best way to find a good hairdresser is to ask someone whose hair you think is stunning who *her* hairdresser is. Even if you have to stop someone on a busy street, subway, or beach to get this information—do it. It's very flattering to be asked this question and no one will mind. The next best way is to check out the fashion magazines for hairstyles you think might translate well on you—and see who is responsible for them.

• If a hairdresser is noted for a particular cut—a trademark—that does not mean the trademark cut will suit you. Be very wary of a hairdresser who tries to inflict his or her trademark on your head.

• If a hairdresser is so opinionated, so sure of himself or herself that your ideas and opinions are treated churlishly—walk out. Do not let that hairdresser's scissors near your head.

• If a hairdresser is a temperamental superstar, above explaining what he or she is doing and why, walk out. Hairdressers like this probably don't know what they are doing and why.

• Just getting a haircut that's in fashion is not enough; you may look terrible in a geometric cut even if that happens to be the current trend. An experienced hairdresser must help you choose a look that's you—and not faddish. Pretty is better than in.

• A good hairdresser should be interested in your life style—to some extent. He or she doesn't need to know your favorite novel but does need to know if you generally need a "dressy" look or a "casual" look, and should be able to give you either in a reasonably maintenance-free cut.

• *Wise words:* Change your hairstylist occasionally. You can always go back. A fresh vision of your hair is worth taking a chance with someone new.

• If your hairdresser, good as he or she is, is too bored, important, or busy to do his or her own work (except for the removal of rollers and clips), walk out. You're not paying to have an apprentice cut and set and comb your hair.

• If you plan to go back, leave a healthy tip. Nothing is quite so inspirational. (If you don't know what a healthy tip is, ask the receptionist what she suggests.)

• If you blow smoke in your hairdresser's face, or have your friends call on his private phone, you get what you deserve: *very* jagged ends.

• If your hairdresser watches himself or herself in the mirror, more than he or she watches you, rethink the hairdresser.

• Finally, a hairdresser who chats incessantly is not paying attention to his or her work. A garrulous barber once asked the ancient Greek philosopher Archelaus how he wished his hair cut. "In silence," replied the philosopher.

My Two Favorite Hair Wizards—
Suga and Richard Stein

They had plenty of wise words for my book. Here are some of the wisest:

SUGA

What's the best brush?

One with a half-synthetic, half-natural bristle. Mason Pearson puts out a good one. For a finished look, a wide-toothed brush or plastic pick also works well. If you have a good cut, just pull out the hair with your fingers—when it's wet; you can even bend the hair with your fingers into the shape you wish.

What should I see in a good cut?

It should fall into place with a shake of the head.

You should not see thickness in one spot, thinness in another.

You should not see pointy places or jagged spots.

You *should* see volume without teasing or spraying.

Should I brush my hair every night? The old one hundred strokes?

No. Massage instead, which is wonderful for circulation and far better for the hair. At shampoo time, think of the wash as a massage for the scalp and pay more attention to the rinse than anything else. Get all that soap *out*.

Can I blow-dry every day?

Yes. You can shampoo and blow-dry daily if you keep the dryer at a moderate heat and move it as you dry each section.

What's a perfect length?

That's hard to say—it differs with each face. One thing's for sure: Long hair tends to drag a woman's face down, and hair should never be longer than shoulder length after forty.

What are some wise words about color?

Never color your hair yourself unless you're experimenting with wash-out, semipermanent color: It will turn out to be disaster. Consider keeping the gray if you're light in complexion; it can be highlighted and frosted to look wonderful.

How often should I cut my hair?

Every three months is minimum. Cut your hair regularly even if you only cut off an eighth of an inch. Hair is not like a tree: It's healthiest at its roots and begins to split farther down the hair shaft.

Are conditioners really helpful?

If you have a permanent, the answer is yes: The hair will dry out rapidly without one. If your hair is untreated, only you can tell, by experimenting, if a conditioner makes it more silky and easy to manage. Cristina uses a protein conditioner after each shampoo, and every couple of weeks she has a heavier, oil-conditioner treatment to counteract the drying, harsh effects of the lights under which she must work.

RICHARD STEIN

• Never decide on a new hair color by yourself: Get a professional opinion from three different hairstylists before you make up your mind.

• The biggest mistake a do-it-yourselfer can make is cutting her own bangs. In the history of the world, it's never worked well.

• A great home rinse for the après shampoo? Try this: one cup water, one tablespoon apple-cider vinegar. Comb through the hair and follow with a clear water rinse. The cider will restore the pH balance to the hair, and the mixture ensures the absence of a soapy film that dulls hair.

• For a great home conditioner, try this: Mix several commercial conditioners (to get the best of each) and bind them with the protein of a beaten egg yolk. Comb through hair and sit under a heat cap (which you can buy in any beauty supply store) or some hot towels. Rinse thoroughly with clear water after fifteen minutes.

• Hair color tip: Any highlights you add ought to be in a shade that's present in your natural hair color. I've brush-painted reddish glints into Cristina's hair because they're natural for her and they look fantastic!

• Tip for black women: Stay far away from the ubiquitous pick. Your hair is exceptionally fragile and you can easily tear or break it. Use your fingers instead.

• Tip for a natural-looking permanent: Ask for a loose body wave.

My Ten Savvy Hair Tips

1. KNOW YOUR BEST LOOK AND DON'T FALL FOR FADS. Sometimes they think bald is cute. Sometimes they think everyone should go Afro. Sometimes they think straight hair is the only way to go. It makes the best sense to go with what looks great on you, what's natural for you, and turn a deaf ear to the "theys"—the hair-fashion pundits. If your hair is naturally curly and you straighten it every few months, you'll be wearing a wig when your hair falls out before you're fifty. Make the most of your hair and don't let the murderers permanent, straighten, tease, and color your hair to death.

2. RINSES ARE NOT FOREVER. No protein, beer, creme, or acid rinse can *permanently* affect the condition, color, or texture of your hair. Rinses can *temporarily* add body to hair or make it easier to style or comb right after a shampoo —and that's all. It doesn't pay to spend a fortune on rinses because their effect is ephemeral. If you use beer, yogurt, mayonnaise, lemon juice, and other kitchen cosmetics in your hair, you'll have icky hair—unless you rinse so many times it becomes terribly boring.

3. SHAMPOOS ARE NOT WHIPPED CREAM. There are currently about five hundred shampoos on the market, with as many esoteric and useless additives. The primary function of a shampoo is to clean. Don't mistake cleaning with the amount of whipped cream lather a shampoo produces: More lather means more detergent, which can be drying and dulling to the hair. Experiment to find the one which cleans best for you. HOT TIP: Even if the manufacturer says you should lather up twice, once is more than enough if you wash your hair every day or so. The real secret to shampooing is in the excellent rinsing, which is vastly more important than the shampoo you choose. For easy combing without a conditioner, try combing your hair while the shampoo is still in: *then* rinse.

4. HAIR THICKENER HYPES. I never met a hair thickener I really liked. Although they seem to give more substance to your hair because they coat each strand with bulk-adding resins, proteins, and other substances, they also leave an unpleasant stickiness, an odd texture. Hair thickeners are a product that can really use some refining.

5. HAIR SPRAYS. Nothing takes the sexiness out of hair faster than a hair spray that creates an armored shield around your head. Run your fingers through such glutinous hair and your fingers are irrevocably trapped.

6. COLORING. Don't do it yourself! Few beauty treatments really need expert care, once you've learned how to do them. Hair coloring is one of the few. And don't go hog wild with color: If your eyebrows are raven, they're going to look tawdry with blond hair. Once you start with coloring, keep it up; different color roots that show are ugly. Highlighting lighter-color hair is a softening thing to do. Highlighting very dark hair with blond tints is almost sure to make it look brassy and cheap. Take your skin tone into consideration before coloring hair: Unless you can really carry it off, very pale skin cannot look terrific with very black hair. Sallow or black skin looks terrible with very light hair. Above all, hair coloring takes time, money, and taste. If you are missing one of the three, stick to your natural color. (Oh, it doesn't take all *that* much money. The other two are absolute necessities.)

7. HAIR TALKS. It does. It has long conversations with people about you. Messy hair says you're a messy thinker. Brash and loudly colored hair tells people you have no sense of style or taste or chic. Boring helmets of the same hairstyle,

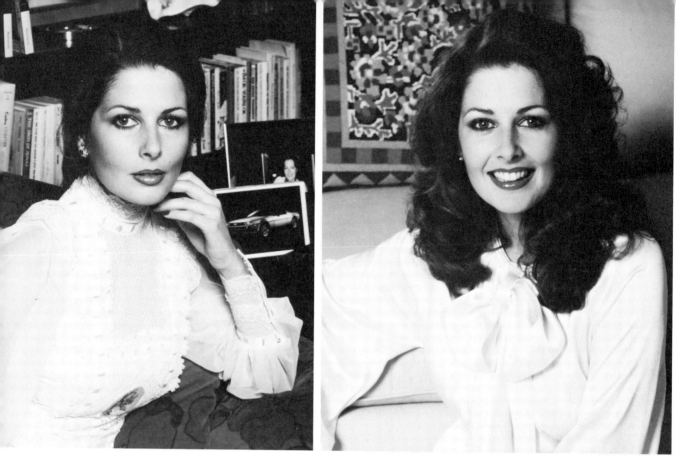

Long hair can hang loose or be sleekened back or up in a variety of styles.

Shorter hair can be clipped back or frizzed into a facial aureole.

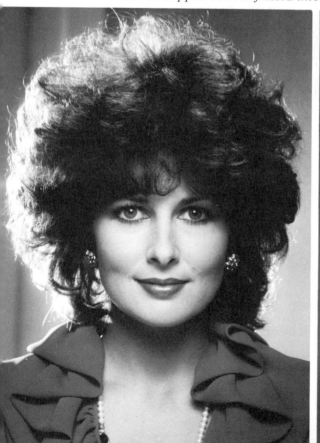

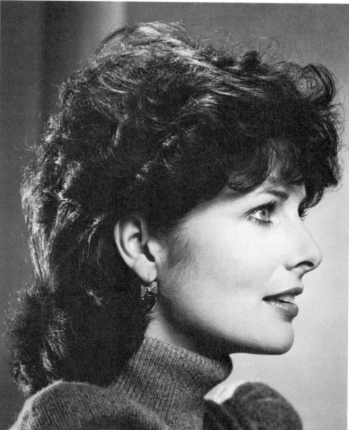

year after year, speak eloquently of your lack of imagination. Springy, clean, soft hair says—you're, well—enchanting. (Funny thing is, it says it even if you're not so enchanting.)

8. KEEP HAIR PRUNED —like a plant, if you will—for maximum strength and attractiveness. A three-inch strand of hair is about six months old, has been shampooed about eighty or ninety times, and has been combed about a hundred and eighty times. It needs pruning or cutting from every six weeks (for very short hair) to every six months for long hair.

9. IGNORE CHARTS that tell you you have to wear your hair in a certain style, depending on the shape of your face. If God had wanted us to always wear our hair the same way because of face shape, it would have been painted on instead of blowing free. The only thing to remember is
- *When it's long,* use the length: Pin it up high in a bun and let the tendrils hang free on the nape of your neck. Or use a comb or a sparkling clip to lift it off your shoulders. Braid it, bunch it, chignon it. Don't spray it into armor. Let the wind toss it around at the beach.
- *When it's short,* sleek it, seal-like, back for tennis or jogging. Wear it asymmetrically one day, slicked back on one side, geometric on the other; curl it so it frizzes into a facial aureole another day.

Whatever style you choose, let it not be middle-aged–Margaret Thatcher style—a sedate, even, all-around look with no shape or flair.

The one style to absolutely avoid is the Curlers-in-the-Supermarket Look. You will never see Jackie Onassis in curlers. Even when she's at Kenneth's, she does it behind a curtain. If you wear curlers in your hair in public, you should be arrested.

10. BUY BARGAINS. Don't get your hair supplies in a beauty salon or a department store. The same supplies can be obtained in a beauty supply shop at discount. Call before you go to make sure the shop is open to the retail-buying public and stock up your supplies of dryers, curlers, hair-care preparations, petroleum jelly (great for coating the hairline before home coloring to prevent a black neck), rubber gloves, sponges—you name it.

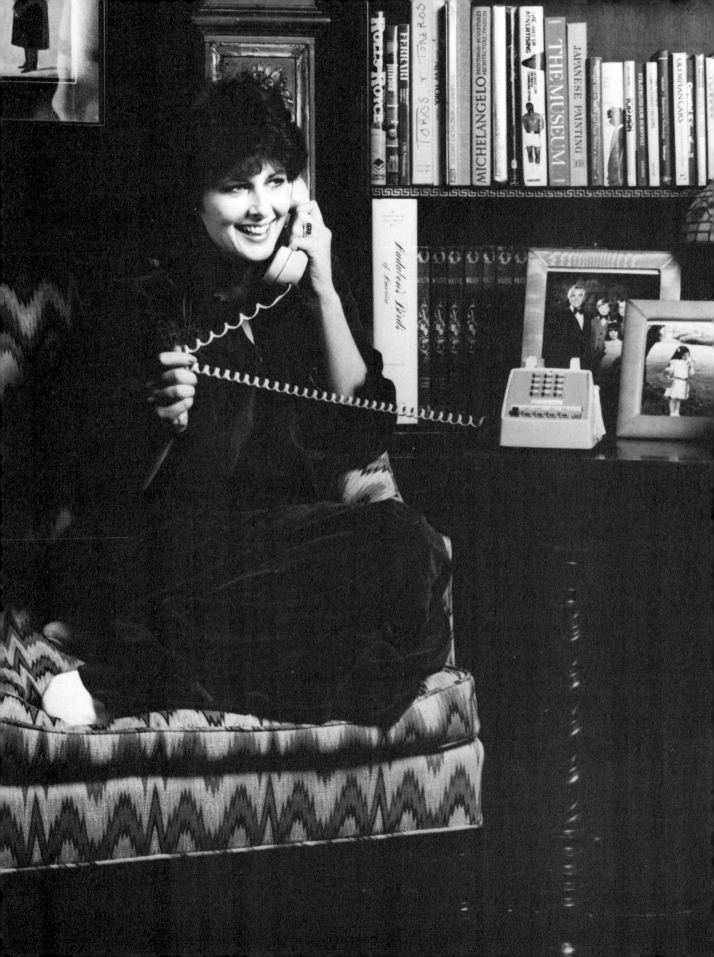

Chapter 5

SELF-STYLE

*I*N the end, style is no more than a presentation of *self*—your inner self, your best self, your most convincing self. We all have those dark nights of the soul when we feel ugly, unloved, or tongue-tied, but the true stylist will wake up in the morning, pinch herself into reality, and primp, pamper, and persuade the best parts of herself to come shining back. That's presentation. When you're looking for a job (or trying to get to the top rung of the one you have), holding forth at a party, attending a business meeting, or walking through your day in a hundred different ways, the way you present yourself, the way you package your assets, determines how successful you'll be. Poise, grace, vitality, and, yes, manners are what make you interesting and appealing. That's the essence of femininity. One of the most misunderstood aspects of the feminist revolution is that people think strong women have to be crass and pushy. Nothing is further from the truth. Politeness and power, charm and integrity, subtlety and strength—are marvelous partners.

Vocal Style

Face, hair, body, and clothes have infinite possibilities for the woman of style. But almost anyone can *look* stylish from afar. The moment she opens her mouth, she gives herself away if she doesn't have self-style. The true test of class is the way a woman sounds—what she says and how she says it. In this chapter, let's talk about talk—and a place where it counts a lot—the workplace.

Your voice and the things you say are clear indicators of style. If you speak in a way that makes people love to listen, your whole image is toned up. Think of voice as another means of power: People react to you much more favorably, give you what you want much more readily, and respect you—yes, *respect* you—more when you have a warm and pleasing speech pattern. You may not be able to make yourself beautiful or rich, but you *can* change your speech style.

Not long ago I was at an elegant party. All of a sudden a hush came over the room. An extraordinary beauty, who shall go nameless here, had just walked in. I'd heard she was quite intelligent also.

Everyone stared. I stared. John stared. She had style written all over her magnificent face, her clothes, her sparkling eyes, her carriage. I tell you, she was really something. Then she spotted someone she knew. He hurried over and whispered something in her ear. She opened her luscious mouth.

"FAYANTAAAS-TIC!" she intoned, nasally. "NO KIDDUN," she whined. You could sense the crowd's surprise. The disappointment in the room was almost palpable. In one minute, this vision had become ordinary. She'd lost her style and even her beauty seemed compromised. I felt embarrassed for her. Everyone at the party lost interest in her.

I think that voice quality and conversational style is probably the most important thing to consider if a woman wishes to leave an impression of grace. If you can speak so that others lust to listen, you've got it made in the shade. Consider the E. F. Hutton advertisement: "When E. F. Hutton talks . . . everyone listens." Clearly that ad wants to convey that E. F. Hutton knows a whole lot about making money, and people who want this information will stop doing just about anything to hear what the guy says. It's an effective ad because it makes sense—people listen to what they wish to hear. But you can take it one step further. A woman with a beautiful speaking voice can make you think that she is about to say something you really *need* to know—even if you really never thought you needed to know it before. A woman with such a voice can lure people into listening to her and, incredible but true, believing her. Her words, even though they're not earth-shattering revelations, sound far more important than they really are. The listener is seduced into believing he's hearing wisdom, originality, sensuality, or sincerity, when he may be hearing nothing of the sort. The fact is that a voice, rich in color and dimension, varying in intensity and low in pitch, *seizes* and *holds* attention and belief. Conversely, a voice that's tinny, raspy, monotonous or slurry, seizes and, just as abruptly, *loses* attention and credulity.

Lauren Bacall, in her autobiography, *Lauren Bacall by Myself*, tells of director Howard Hawks as he spoke with her, an unknown eighteen-year-old actress.

Hawks told Bacall that most women tended to raise their voices when they got excited and advised her to train her own voice to remain low and resonant.

And so she did. "I found a spot on Mulholland Drive and proceeded to read aloud, keeping my voice lower and louder than normal. If anyone had ever passed by, they would have found me a candidate for an asylum. Who sat on mountaintops in cars reading books aloud to the canyons? I did."

She got the part. *To Have and Have Not* with her soon-to-be husband, Humphrey Bogart, made that woman and that voice immortal. "If you want me, just whistle," the voice, deep, throbbing, sexy murmured—and no one forgot it.

There are two major factors to a beautiful speaking voice, and they are the sound of the voice and diction. Diction includes the choice of words and the distinctness of your pronunciation. And both are in your power to change. I've said that style is an acquired art. So is a great voice. Everyone, unless you're born with a vocal cord or mouth abnormality, is capable of voice control. You can develop poor habits of tonality and diction—but you can improve them. Check the following list, and be honest: Are any of these speaking disasters *your* speaking disasters?

FILLERS. You know what I mean. I mean, uh, I mean. You know, You know. Ummmm. I mean. And-uh, *then*.

SPEAKING WITH A LITTLE-GIRL, HIGH-PITCHED TONE. Try getting a job with this kind of voice which says, "I'm just a little kid and *hate* to be out of my playroom." You have a little girl voice if, when answering the phone, anyone has ever asked to speak to your daddy.

SPEAKING WITH A WHINE OR A TWANG. It says you'd be great out on the ranch but a misery to live with.

SPEAKING WITH A HARSH, GRATING SOUND —like chalk scraped on a blackboard. Forget going to the audition.

SPEAKING MONOTONOUSLY. You say, "Oh, rub me *there*, darling" in the same tone of voice with which you say, "My feet hurt."

SPEAKING WITHOUT R's. Or too harsh G's. Or no I's. Or something else. Regional dialects can be charming if they're not caricatures. New Yawwwk. LonGG GIsland. Vanella ice cream. If you ignore or crudely exaggerate certain letters of certain words, they come out giving you a very deflated image.

MUMBLING. Blubba lova blurpin huvva vuv.

It may be that you don't recognize any of the above. Listen to yourself on tape. You really don't know what your voice sounds like because it changes as it leaves your mouth. Assume, if you have a good tape recorder, that what you hear when you play back your voice is what others hear. Then be honestly critical. (HINT: Tape yourself as you talk on the phone so you get an accurate idea of speech patterns. If you make a recording just for analysis, you'll be too careful and not really yourself.)

If you hate the way you sounded on tape, if you meant to be firm and you came across sounding angry, if you meant to be sexy and you came across sounding stupid, if you meant to be soft and lulling and you came across sounding strident—do something about it. Here are some things you can do:

1. Go to the library and get a book on speaking effectively. This is something you really can teach yourself.

2. If you would rather work with a professional, look in the Yellow Pages for one, listed under "Speech," or "Voice," or "Communication."

In the meantime, here are some workable suggestions to try:

FOR A MONOTONOUS VOICE: Read out loud with *expression* as your second-grade teacher used to urge. Change your tone, shade your adjectives, make your verbs *move* with meaning.

FOR A TOO LOW OR TOO LOUD VOICE: Practice sending it out to different parts of the room. Talk to three feet away, then six feet away, until you get accustomed to varying levels needed for distances.

FOR DROPPING LETTERS AND MURDERING OTHERS: Exaggerate or *explode* the letters you're missing, for a while. PERRRRRfectly. New YoRRRRRRk. If you're too hard on certain letters (LonGGG GIsland instead of Long Island), soften the offending sounds by having your tongue meet the palate very gently instead of tightly. Don't force sounds—blend them softly. Splendid. Not splendiDDD.

FOR A LITTLE-GIRL VOICE: Relax. Put your voice way down in your throat so it sounds fuller, more resonant. Practice saying *ng* sounds softly, deeply, keeping that pitch *low* (sing, ring, ping . . .).

FOR MUMBLES: Stick a pencil in your mouth sideways and say "Peter Piper Picked a Peck of Pickled Peppers." Open your mouth when you speak. *Shape* your lips around *wh, th, m, f, b* sounds. That's enunciation.

The Things You Say

Voice is one thing: What you say is quite another. It has always seemed to me quite miraculously appealing when a woman has a *living*, colorful vocabulary. That means avoiding slang like "ya know?" "like it's heavy, man," "the thing about it is . . . " It's hard to make a stunning presentation of self if you sound like an illiterate. Learn a word a day (don't bury it in an old schoolbook—*use* it); use colorful interesting words (*canary* instead of *yellow*, *glisten* instead of *shine*). Wake up your conversation with animated and provocative language.

And avoid euphemisms—those words that skip around the subject (if you've had a face lift, it's not a cosmetic reorganization; dying is not passing on).

The Things You Don't Say

Verbal presentation sometimes is as much a matter of silence as language. Listen. It takes two to make a conversation—anything less is a speech. Don't interrupt, yet you don't have to wait impatiently till it's your turn to talk. Conversation can be touches also. A radiant smile, a squeeze of a hand, intense eye contact—all speak poetry. The human touch says more than convoluted speech. And sometimes a brief grasp of a listener's hand calls attention to what your mouth is saying.

Self-style is not being rude. Even to surly taxi drivers, skeptical salespeople, arrogant waiters; you can feel *sorry* for them and think they're creeps, but keep your cool and your class. Style is not being hostile when you've been caught doing a wrong or not-nice thing (apologizing is *huge* style). Style is not being stuffy when the joke's on you.

Self-Presentation in the Workplace

Self-style is important when you wake up and face your husband, when you circulate at the cocktail party, and when you go to the PTA meeting, but perhaps it is most important in the workplace. If you care about making it in a career, you'd better make sure your inner class shines through when you're dealing with bosses, clients, and coworkers. And that's true for any job at all. The trappings may change, the job descriptions may differ, the products may not even resemble each other—but the success style in almost every workplace remains the same. The principles, the rules of the game, are constant no matter if you make cars, dresses, computers, or beautiful faces. I'm a model and I've always been one, but I have noticed through the years that my friends in other professions who are equally successful act the same way I do in the workplace. That doesn't mean we are carbon copies of each other. It means that Upward Mobility generally understands the unwritten laws—and that's work style. There are exceptions of course —the man who is crass, rude, and boorish—*and* successful; the woman who is sloppy, arrogant, and unpunctual—*and* is still successful. But they are few and far between. I've talked with many experts successful in different areas of business (and I know from my own accomplishments in *my* business) about the un-

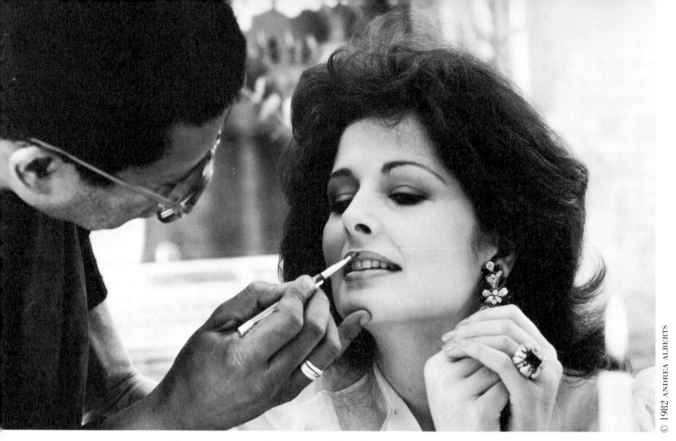

Cooperation and a smile add professionalism and warmth. Here I am with makeup artist Joey Mills.

written laws of work style—and I'll tell you just what they are in a moment. First, allow me some generalities on the subject.

Generally speaking, I deeply believe that consideration, politeness, good manners are the most effective way to bring style to the work arena. There are many exquisite women in the world who could be dynamite models, but who never receive that "call back"; I assume that's true in other professions as well, where talented people somehow just miss the boat. That's because, in the real world, Joan Crawford–type superstars don't cut it anymore. It's talent and attitude—not aura. I attribute my own success to my conviction that people need to be recognized, paid respect—not catered to but *listened* to. By listening, I don't mean obeying—I mean *listening.* How many times have you spoken to someone whose attention was riveted just beyond your left ear, waiting for the more important person to enter the room? I find that the height of crass. In the famous Arthur Miller play *Death of a Salesman,* Willy Loman's wife tells her son that, to their father, "*attention must be paid.*" I try to pay attention to the people with whom I work by being totally professional. By politeness. By always being on time for appointments. By being considerate of their requests. You may hear that people in the acting or modeling professions are "princesses" who have little respect for others' timetables, but I'll tell you, every *thorough* professional I've ever met, no matter how glitzy or glamorous her reputation, shows up for work on time and does her job creditably. Princesses don't last long when they're not royalty. It can't hurt to be thoughtful in small ways, either. To bring a small gift to a coworker whose son has just graduated. To send a card for a job well done. To ask, in a way that shows you want to hear the answer, how someone's sick wife is.

And another generality but one that always seems to ring true: The person who is true to her nature and to her individuality is the one that inevitably rises to the top. The job should bear the stamp of your special personality—you don't become the job. Take my friend Cheryl Tiegs. She came to modeling at a time when bouffant haircombs, exaggerated makeup, and sophisticated glamour was the rage. But Cheryl was all clean faced, easygoing, California laid-back. She refused to conform—and became one of the most sought-after models in the business. Conrad Hilton ignored the fad of el-cheapo, thrift-type motels and stuck to his style of big, expensive, and glossy. Hilton makes a lot of money. Gloria Steinem is a glamorous feminist who has often been accused of "selling out" because she cares about fashionable hairstyle and attractive eyeglasses. On the contrary, she has done more for feminism than any braless, dowdy, strident spokesperson. Princess Di is bringing her style of chic and modern to a royalty noted for frumpiness—and it hasn't done her or the royal image any harm at all. The workplace has room for your special brand of humor, aggressiveness, and standards. You don't have to be macho to be a successful man, and you don't have to be fluttery to be a successful woman: You just have to be *you*.

On the other hand, you can't overdo individuality either. You are not required to swim in the pool (whether it be the secretary pool or the top executive pool), but then again, if you do swim, you can't swim nude. You have to be aware of others' sensibilities as well as your own style.

Let me give you an example in my own workplace and work life where I did what I had to, even though it wasn't the norm—and still came out on top.

Models are supposed to be at the whim of the client, photographer, agency, and magazine editors . . . when working. I can understand the need for such professionalism. Nevertheless, my family has always come first and if my child has a sore throat and temperature, I *will* call home twenty times, I will check out her status—no matter if it keeps Scavullo, Way Bandy, Eileen Ford, and *Vogue* all waiting. I will *not* accept jobs that keep me away from home, on location, for long periods of time. I always stop a shoot around three to make sure my son has gotten home from school. And you know what? Except for occasional grumbling, everyone accepts it. They know there can be no negotiation on certain points. In return, I am absolutely the best model, the most responsible and caring person working in my field—I *am!* But my style came before anything—and that was okay.

What follows are the rules that *can't* be broken as well as ways to bring style and success to *any* work arena.

1. GET MAD. If you hate the way something is being done, march into the boss's office and tell him or her. Let your energy, your passion carry you. Speak in a low voice, but speak in exclamation marks. Make sure you have some concrete suggestions on how to *fix* the thing you hate. Complaints without solutions are wearisome and unhelpful. Your impetuous move may just get you a raise; bosses like aggressive style.

2. QUESTION MEDIOCRITY. If something is just okay—don't accept it for a minute. The work you turn out, the ideas you offer in your workplace should be consistently *fine*, not average. Not just acceptable. If your style is recognized as one that accepts only top-banana work and ideas, your workplace will come to shine.

3. DON'T BE AFRAID OF HUMOR. Inevitably the kid who gets accepted to the best college is the one who made the interviewer laugh. The woman who makes the most points with clients and with the boss is the one who sees humor in life—and allows herself to share it with those she works with. Not the lampshade-on-the-head or the joke-telling kind of humor, but the kind of wit that laughs at itself, that makes bosses human—and shows them you like them and they don't terrify you. Humor is heady stuff.

4. IF YOU'RE IN A DEAD-END JOB, recognize it. Then get rid of it. A woman of style almost always refuses a powerless position—one which places her at the mercy of everyone else's imagination. And don't be terrorized of temporary joblessness; it can change your life for the better.

5. DON'T LET THE BOSS scare the pants off you. Style in the workplace *depends* on your recognizing your worth to him or her. Undue subservience to others gives *them* strength—not you. Keep your head up, and your kow-towing down—even if the president of the company is in the general area. Remember: Presidents also get pimples on their noses, runs in their stockings, and cramps.

6. ENTERTAIN THEM ON YOUR TURF. But make your turf classy. There's no rule you can't have your boss, peers, and associates to your home for dinner/cocktails/good talk. That creates a new atmosphere at work—one that's in your favor. However, no "bring-your-own-bottle" parties, no potluck parties, no cheap dinnerware, no "everybody-come-in-jeans" invitations. Make no mistake: Unless your business associates are your real pals, you're still "working" at a home party—just in a different location. Don't do it if you can't do it with style.

7. DO THE EXECUTIVE STRUT. The look of confidence in your walk, talk, and dress gives you confidence—and gives everybody else confidence in *you*. Stand straight. Don't slouch over your desk. Never go to work wearing something you hate, something that undermines your attractiveness or your security "blanket." Never go to work in anything torn, stained, or pinned. (You can't do an executive strut if your under- or overpinnings are coming loose.)

8. STOP APOLOGIZING SO MUCH. Accept yourself and your frailties.

Don't always seek acceptance from others or ego massage. Before you apologize for things said or actions taken, say to yourself, "Am I *really* sorry?" If not, zip your lip. Apologizing constantly is not stylish.

9. DON'T BE EVERYONE'S BEST FRIEND. Style in the workplace does not mean confiding in a business associate about your homosexuality, your poverty problems, or your son's hostility. It makes people uncomfortable. It's not appropriate. It undermines your professional status. The people you work with didn't choose you as their closest and dearest pal and, therefore, don't have to be burdened with your hot opinions on politics or your personal life style. It sounds unfriendly and even a little bit snobbish to say all this, but intimacy is simply out of place at work.

10. DON'T BE AN EXTREMIST. Being a woman of style at work allows you to be an individual but doesn't include being *flamboyantly* different. While that may be interesting to your lover and even your mother—it is inappropriate in the workplace. Extreme means wearing bizarre or trendy clothing. Smoking fat cigars if you're a woman. Talking a lot about your two lovers with whom you live. Being militant about anything. I'm not saying, at all, that you have to quash your feelings about, say, inequal pay for women and blacks: I just say you shouldn't hand out pamphlets at the office.

11. BE POLITE. I think this is the heavy one. Politeness and respect for others doesn't mean subservience. If you're going to be late, telephone and advise those who are waiting. If you have inadvertently trod on someone's psyche, don't just let it pass—explain yourself and offer your apologies. (Here is where an apology *is* in order.) Politeness and consideration toward others are professional attributes.

12. FINALLY, LEARN HOW TO COMMAND ATTENTION IN AN ELEGANT MODE. You don't have to beg, kick, or scream to avoid being ignored. In a restaurant, don't flutter your hands or shriek for the waiter. *Lower* your voice and call him firmly but with dignity. Never wait *too* long for any appointment (more than half an hour is too long). When kept hanging, you quietly tell a receptionist you have five minutes more of waiting time and then will leave . . . and you do. You make it clear by your quiet dignity (and by asking, not hinting for attention) that you're a valuable person.

It's reassuring to know that in the workplace as well as in dress, makeup, furnishing, and relationships, style is almost always an acquired art. That is, if you don't have it, there are places to learn it. All kinds of programs are available to teach you how to build up an effective business persona, whether it's in the area of your speech, dress, assertiveness, or personality. Whether you like the word or not, often it's your packaging that counts in the workplace. The little jewel that's you, inside, is often neglected or lost to vision if the style of the gift wrap—the outside—reads second class.

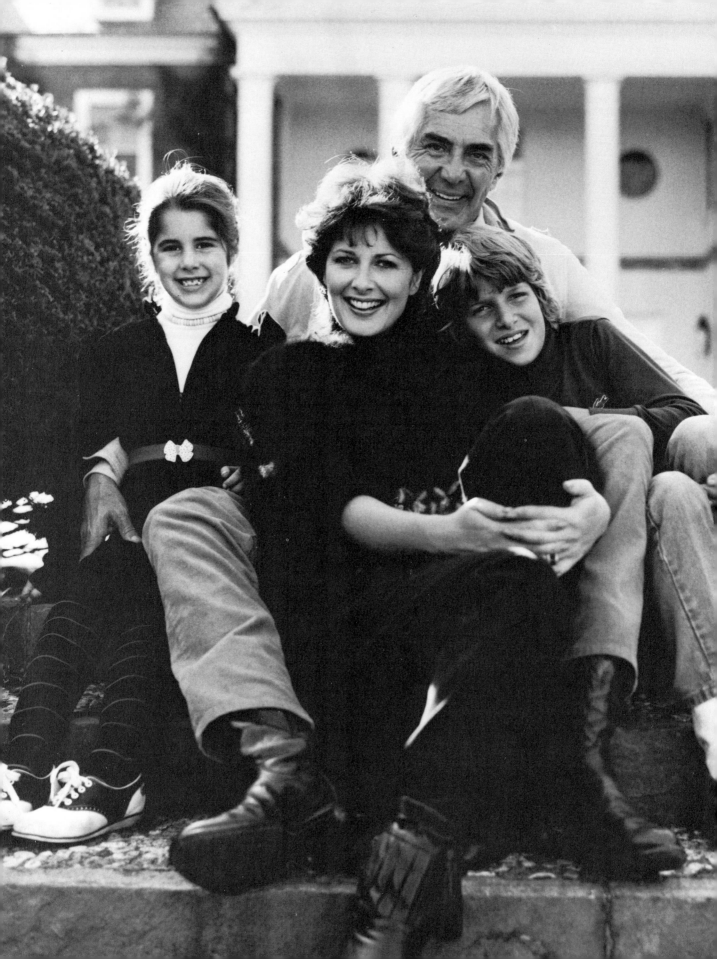

Chapter **6**

PEOPLE STYLE

*T*HERE'S style in clothing, face, and figure—and make no mistake—there's high style in relationships. I call it people style. The way you are with your mate, friends, and family reflects your style in the most telling way. Have you ever seen a stunning woman verbally abusing her children in the supermarket? Or the same stunning woman being cuttingly sarcastic to her husband at a party? It kind of takes away from "stunning"—to say the least. It's not just appearances I'm speaking of. Your whole presence, psyche, inner self is reflected in the way you are with the people to whom you are closest. Let's begin with . . .

Love Style

Men and women together are more than sensualists. They're (if they're doing it right) true buddies, imagination-sparkers, and loyalists. Unfortunately, in love relationships, unstylish players invariably show up. Four of the worst are:

THE OVERLAPPER

She hangs all over her lover, sits on his lap at parties, gets lipstick on his collar and nose, tickles his thigh in public. She's a definite turnoff, a woman who reads *needy* instead of *seductive*.

MS. GOOD-TIME CHARLOTTE

She gives him presents, massages his ego, says flattering things to his friends and boss, but she doesn't understand loyalty and commitment. She's ready for the roller-coaster ride when it's on the upswing, but the moment the trip takes a downward turn, she wants off. She'll love him as long as he's rich, handsome, or powerful, but watch out on the sharp turns.

THE SAINT

She's boring. She's never concerned with her own importance; she plays down her preferences and needs and dehumanizes herself. "Oh, whatever you want to do is fine with me. No, of course I don't mind waiting outside in this hailstorm." Such a love style has no panache!

THE LESSER HALF

Related to the Saint, the Lesser Half doesn't only play down her needs—she *submerges* them in her partner's ego, life, or world so completely that she has no ego, life, or world of her own. She waits for him to come home to enliven her day because she has no day of her own worth speaking of. It's important to walk your own stride because no one loves to love a mirror image of himself. Whether your work is in the home or in the office, do it creatively: enlarge your interests and talents so you're no one's Lesser Half.

Why do so many love relationships fade or need outside stimulation? I'm convinced that it's because people who are married for a few years seem to stop trying to be wonderful. They take each other for granted—a fatal flaw. They don't do any of the seductive things they did before marriage like tease, flirt, touch. It's a shame. Relationships and marriages can be renewed time and time again by having *expectations*, by expecting the other to be the romantic, exciting person to whom you were once drawn. He was there once, that person who covered you up in the middle of the night, brought champagne to celebrate your eyes, loved to take showers with you. That same person is still there—waiting for you to rediscover his essential self that seems to have gotten lost through the years. Finding him again is the most stylish thing you can do for your love. People are always amazed at "the new man" that emerges when a divorced man finds a new love. He's not new at all—he's been there all the time, but his wife lost sight of that part of him.

If *expecting* to find a terrific person in your lover is important, so is *accepting*. None of us stays nubile, twenty-four, and firm. If you feel like a failure or make your partner feel like one because of more weight and less money than either of you hoped for, that sense of failure colors your entire self-perception. It tends to make you act negatively. People who are most successful in intimate relationships are those who are not judgmental because the other doesn't live up to perfection.

Another rule of the game, as far as I'm concerned, is monogamy. I know that sounds old-fashioned, but despite all the fads about open marriage and sexual playmates I could not exist in a marriage that accepts sexual relations with other partners. Sure, I've been attracted to other men during the twelve years we've been together, but an affair would be too dangerous a chance to take: It would *have* to take the edge off our mutual trust, and our relationship could never again be quite the same. I don't think I could be happy in even a relationship, let alone a marriage, that allowed varying sexual partners. Being each other's best friend, for me, implies not experimenting with others. Nothing is ever perfect: Bodies have flaws and so do lives, and true bonding means commitment. That's *my* sense of love style.

Styles differ and, surely, so do orchestrations of love relationships, but in every successful one I ever heard of, there seem to be three givens that are consistently present. They are:

• Taking the time to be together, to talk, to walk, to read, to just Be. Every moment doesn't have to be a tennis match or a theater appointment or dinner with friends.

• Letting each other know what feels good, what makes you happy. Mind reading is not part of the marriage covenant.

• Not being judgmental. Judging and criticizing are sure erotica dampeners. Acceptance and growing together breed love.

And then there's friendship with its joys and obligations and also, I'm afraid, limitations. Let me tell you about my own . . .

Friend Style

I'll be frank. My feeling about friends has changed drastically since our lives became the stuff of headlines all over the world. Before the "troubles" I would have died for my friends, and I assumed they would have done the same for me. But I suppose it takes a tragedy to find certain kinds of truths and the truth with many of those friends was that they were along for the ride as long as John and I provided glamour and laughs; the moment we needed support, the moment we were down—many friends deserted the ship. Which makes me, I think, an even greater authority on style in the art of friendship—because, make no mistake, friendship is an art that cries out for style. What I am about to say is controversial, I understand, but it is important that I say it anyway.

I firmly believe that even the closest of friends, the dearest of comrades, must respect a delicate balance in their friendship that can, with a wrong word or a misunderstood bit of advice, turn suddenly sour. The gift of friendship is a very sensitive act. The truest, most cherished friends I have are those I love deeply—but I still would not confide my *most* intimate thoughts to them. Because (although it may sound cold) a friend is not a husband, not a daughter, not a mother or father, not a sister or brother. It is my feeling that although it is superb to share with friends, it is not fair to share your most personal secrets with them. It is rarely appreciated when you burden your friends with intimacies about your life they may not be able to handle. The more secrets your friend tells you, the more guarded you have to be about keeping them, the more vulnerable your relationship grows. What's more, there may come a time when your friend, as much as she loves you, may feel resentful that you carry such power in your hands. It is power, you know, knowing everything about someone else; and that power can easily be abused on purpose or even by accident.

Let me give you an example: When my husband was arrested, I turned to my friend who knew every innermost secret detail about the relationship I had with my husband. She felt she had to protect *her* husband, her family, from scandal. She turned her back. I'd give anything in the world to have our spoken intimacies back safe with me again. I turned to another friend, a loyal and good one, who risked her family's social status to cling to our friendship. She was wonderful, she was loyal—but I needed even more. I needed her total *grief*. She could not, of course, give that much to me. She had her own life to lead—her work, her own luncheon appointments, beauty parlor arrangements, teacher conferences to keep. Of course, she did. And I understand. But I felt sorry I'd given her so huge a part of me and my husband. It seemed, in retrospect, unnecessary.

So it is my feeling now that friendship is to be held dear but not abused with overintimacies. One saves those for one's family. Of course, there is that rare, that extraordinary, that one-in-a-million friendship where sisterhood is not just a term; for that unique, peerless friend whose agony is yours and yours is hers in every sense of the word—let go. Otherwise, share joys, share sorrows, but, it seems to me, keep some part of yourself and your life private. That is the way to make and keep a friend in the real world. One can, you know, with a good and true friend, *listen* to her unspoken needs—and respond to them. Style in friendship is not having to spell everything out.

Having said that, let me tell you what I think *does* make for style in a splendid friendship—besides spilling your guts—all of them:

ACCEPT YOUR FRIEND'S STYLE. Being judgmental spells sure death for friendship. If someone does things differently from you—keep your lecture to yourself. I learned not to interfere with my best friend's style, even though I disapproved of many things she did. Once I told her how I felt and we had the most traumatic argument—it was worse than breaking up with a lover, far worse. I never did it again.

EXPECT LOYALTY. Give it and expect it back. If you're not getting it, it's not friendship.

LISTEN. Eyes riveted on your friend when she speaks. Total attention.

Meaningful responses. You can't have a friend who listens to your *schtick* if you don't listen to hers.

BE THERE FOR HER. When she travels, be there to say goodbye and to greet her when she gets back. When she's ready to kill her children, take them for an overnight visit. If she has a birthday, make her a party, make her a cake, make her a gesture of love.

TOUCH HER. In America, we've forgotten how to touch. In my parents' country, Italy, men know how to caress other men, women hug their best friends and hold hands with them while walking . . . without funny looks. It's wonderful. I embrace my friends, hold them, let them know I care.

GIVE GIFTS. Finally, the art of gift giving is one to cultivate in any friendship of true style. I treasure the gifts my friends have given me over the years; it is a symbol of love to give a gift.

MY FAVORITE GIFTS

Let me tell you some of the gifts I enjoy giving to my friends: gifts that are given "for no special reason" are the most appreciated ones of all because they have the surprise element added to the caring thought. A wonderful plant, a fabulous French casserole dish, a whole wheel of cheese, a bottle of Dom Perignon, a message in chocolate. This last is always a welcome gift and there are many fine chocolate shops that specialize in chocolate in meaningful shapes. Someone sent me a giant aspirin made of chocolate when John's arrest was giving me a major heartache—not to mention headache. Hand-embroidered pillows that my friends have given me occupy a special place in my home. An antique "anything" is a wonderful gift simply because even the person who has everything surely doesn't have it. Homemade jams or jellies or fruit in clear and shining Mason jars are greatly appreciated, as is imported mustard in a wonderful ceramic crock. For an anniversary or an engagement, two Baccarat crystal wineglasses to toast each other. A game of Monopoly. Fifty velvet ribbons for someone who wears her hair tied with a ribbon. (Somehow, giving a simple object in a huge quantity makes it terrific—a ten pound sack of peanuts is a *great* gift. So is a crate of grapes.)

You get the idea. Friends of great style give gifts in style—none of those silver toothpicks, those boxes of handkerchiefs which are tasteless and lacking in *zest*.

I love to feed my friends. Food is one of the most loving, nurturing gifts in the world, and cooking something with joy is a gesture of the deepest affection. Bringing food to the hospital is an especially welcome gift since most hospital food is disaster. When my friend Eileen had surgery, there was my very best osso bucco to greet her. She says she never heard of osso bucco before that day, but all wrapped up with a pretty ribbon, she never forgot its message: "I love you—feel better."

Gifts that are personal and show *thought* are never forgotten. Sure, I could have brought my friend a bottle of perfume or a pretty blouse from a trip I took, but bringing her a baseball cap with a huge parrot that resembles her own talking parrot went over much bigger. (Actually, I hate her dumb parrot, but she doesn't—so the gift was meaningful.) A personal gift you might give to make an older person feel like a VIP is a card from the President: If you know someone who is eighty or older or has a fiftieth or more years' anniversary, write the Greetings Office of the White House, Washington, D.C. 20500, and tell them the full name, address, occasion being celebrated, and date four weeks in advance of the occasion to receive such a card.

Parents and Kids

Style doesn't stop with friends and lovers. It should live within the bond that was once the closest of all—mother and father and the kids.

I've learned that, as in all else, the finest way to deal with these relationships is to be yourself. That means thinking for yourself. Let me give you an example: In almost every current child-care book, one reads the words, "What's valuable is not the quantity of time you spend with kids but the quality of that time." Not true. Quality counts, but boy, so does quantity. I'm the original working mother and no one can accuse me of not being a modern, liberated woman, but I believe that family life can be intact only if you put in the hours. That doesn't mean not working outside the home; what it means, if possible, is working the hours your kids are in school and being there as soon as possible, afterward. It means taking them with you, if possible, and calling regularly, if not possible. If you must be away at work, make the effort of taking the children to see where it is so they can identify and place you in familiar surroundings when you are gone. (Many businesses today have provided for child care right on the premises, and that's always wonderful.) It takes a huge effort to spend the physical hours raising your kids, trying to make them quality hours as well. The point of view that you have to leave young people totally alone, give them leeway and privacy without question, is just wrong. I think it's crucial to know what's happening in their lives—all the time. That doesn't mean you don't respect a closed door; it just means you have a good idea of what's happening behind the door.

I love my children with the most enormous intensity. They make me feel happy and contented and they know I'm rarely far away. I have to work, but they feel the long arm of mother through the telephone many times a day, and through my physical presence *whenever* it's possible.

My own parents were always there. I can't remember ever being alone until I was a pretty grown-up teenager. That may seem smothering by today's standards, but for me, it provided a cement bonding that has always given me support. The world today is moving toward its "freedom" from family ties and responsibilities. To me, freedom is in the knowledge that no matter what happens, you can absolutely depend on your family.

There's a lot of lip service given to roots. Well, roots aren't just there; they're not rigid. They need nourishment and room to flex. You have to treat roots with respect. These are some of the ways my children, my parents, and I try to do that:

EVERYONE NEEDS A CHEERING SECTION. A loving family will give importance to each member. The friends, school, and fun of my daughter, Kathryn, are taken very seriously. She horseback rides like a champion at five, and her *whole* family is always there to cheer her on at meets. Every stage of her growing up is taken seriously. Her needs are respected. Her burgeoning sexuality is respected (yes, even five year olds are sexual creatures). And both children are encouraged to be independent. They remind me of the deer who visits us daily at our country house. Although he's quite wild, he took to coming so often for food and loving we ended up putting a collar on him to alert hunters to stay away. Our kids and that lovely deer are all free spirits who keep coming back for fixes of love and nurturing.

Zach, at twelve, is growing into a young man. We talk about his adolescent yearnings, the things he fears—whatever; it's important always to *talk!* He was adopted when he was very young. Sometimes he needs a little extra reassurance because he's such a gentle, sensitive person. I recently made him his very own photograph album that started with pictures of John's and my wedding. "I was already born when my parents got married—that's how special *I* am," reads the caption. "I'm the famous DeLorean kid, you see. . . ." In every way, I reinforce Zach's individuality when I can. Recently, the two of us, sans sister and Daddy, just took off to Epcot Center (part of Disney World in Orlando, Florida) where we went on rides, stayed up late, and talked about girls for a whole weekend.

OUR PARENTS. My own parents are wonderful. Sometimes they seem rigid about their views, and I've learned to control my temper and my need to always win arguments. It's easier for me to bend than they, I figure. Every woman is a daughter—every father a son. Our experiences are repeated and shared through the years. Vital and independent sons and daughters spring from understanding the pain and joy of their own parents. The huge style of my own parents lies in their respect for us, whether we do it their way or our way.

I guess the essence of what I believe to be style in parent-child relationships is that no one is always just one or the other. In every mother is the memory of her own childhood—the young girl she was is still very much with her. And in every child is the potential of adulthood, parenthood, and somewhere in him or her is that primordial knowledge. No one ever has to be *all* grown up or *all* kid. Sometimes my kids have the most mature, wisest insights. And sometimes I act in an absolutely adolescent manner. What's important is that each lets the other be many things.

One more absolute in the parent–child relationship: It's not a sin to *need* each other. Sometimes in this modern society, we're made to feel guilty for not being absolutely independent. How blessed to be needed and to need others. And how great to be able to forgive our families and ourselves for not being perfect.

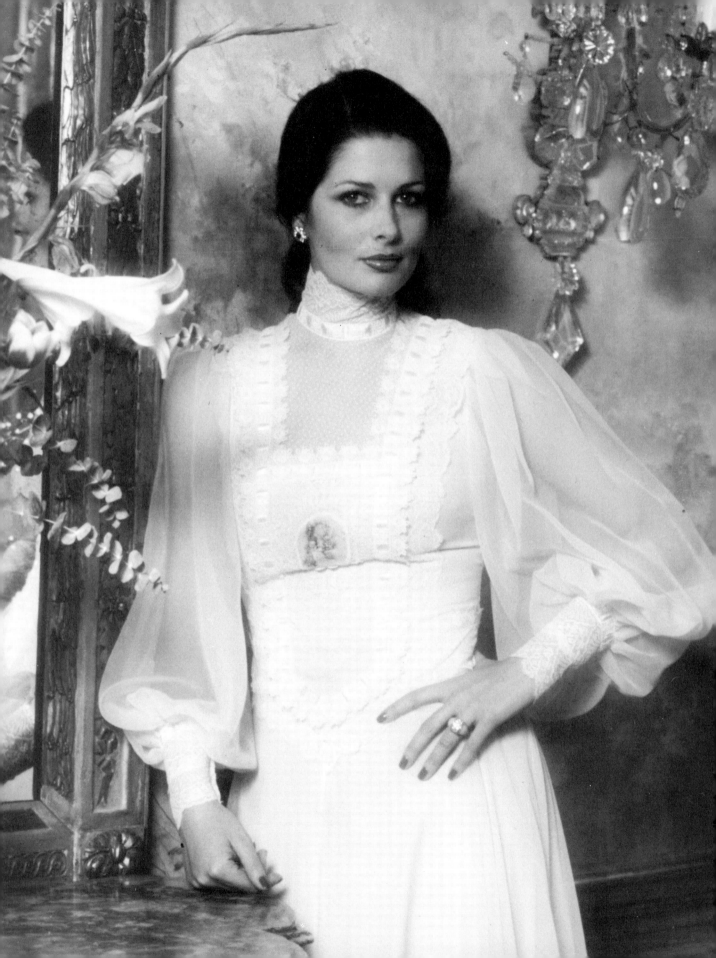

Chapter 7

HOME STYLE

*Y*OU should like to go home.

If ever there was a place where you ought to feel loved and lovable—it should be your home, whether that home takes up two rooms or twenty. For me, there are three essential requisites of home. A home should be:

1. COMFORTABLE. My home is my nest, my resting place. As Robert Frost once said about home, it's the place where "when you go there, they have to take you in." What's more, it should *work*. My home provides me with the functional places and appliances I need to be healthy, creative with food, and generally playful. In that way, it's something like a machine I have come to depend on.

2. INVITING LOOKING. It's my showplace. I bring into my home those people in the world for whom I care, and I show it off because I'm proud of the way it beckons.

3. REPRESENTATIVE OF ME. A home should express the personality of those who live there. It should include those "things" that seem full of wonder and beauty to its inhabitants. It should be an environment that sparks the same delight and response you hope *you* spark in other people. It should have a stamp of individuality about it.

I put my home *around* me in much the same way that I do my clothes, my friends, and my family . . . and so it better be comfortable and pleasing. If you've ever gone to the theater and seen a stage set that surrounds the characters that seems artificial and stiff, you've noticed that the play and the characters also seem to ring false—that's how important a set designer is. The paintings, the furniture, the colors, the objects with which we surround ourselves in our homes better be true to our own instincts or else the environment seems clumsy.

By that I mean:

• Don't display the tiny figurines your mother-in-law gave you for your last anniversary if you *hate* tiny figurines (even if you *love* your mother-in-law). They will yell *her* style, not yours.

• Don't line your bookcases with civil war tomes, Shakespearean sonnets, or feminist manifestos unless you read them.

• Don't display poor reproductions of the "real things" you can't afford. It's far better to have one or two real paintings, real objets d'art and a lot of empty space than a room cluttered with junky imitations. Your home should be uniquely *you*. There has never been anyone quite like you before—and there never will be. That authenticity, that originality, should be reflected in your home. Unless, of course, you are a copycat by true nature—in which case, the poor imitations *will* be you.

It seems to me, then, that the best way to think of your home is as an extension of yourself which reverberates as clearly in the decoration of your turf as it does in the decoration of your physical person. Style flows on to your environment.

Someone once asked the late, great jazz musician Fats Waller, "What is swing?" He replied, "Boy, if you gotta ask, you ain't got it." The same does *not* go for style. You *should* ask, you should do research. Just as you don't have to be born with a "clothes sense," you don't have to be born with a "house sense." Read the decorating magazines until you sense what's elegant and what's ugly in the minds of the professionals—and then adapt their ideas to *your* taste. Go to the model rooms in the department stores, and check out the homes of your friends whose personal and clothing styles you admire. Keep your eyes open, keep a notebook to jot down ideas, and think of it as fun—not drudgery.

Just as it doesn't take a fortune of money to dress yourself with class and style, it doesn't take a fortune to decorate your home. What it does take is a strong voice—your family's voice. Not the decorator's. Not your Aunt Flo's from Hohokus who bequeathed you her shooting gallery shepherdess collection. Style in the *real* world doesn't need a million-dollar investment or decorator because good taste cannot be all that good if it's not *your* taste. I have, of course, many friends who opt for the most renowned decorators to "do" their homes, and, of course, everything always comes out just beautifully. No one can fault a Billy Baldwin or a Mark Hampton sense of elegance. There's never (well, hardly ever) a wrong note in these homes. The only trouble is that each of these homes could easily belong to anyone else with great wealth; the only signature to the design is the decorator's. I think it's a mistake and not the essence of style. Take, for example, one good friend. Unlike me, she was born with the proverbial silver spoon in her mouth. My father was a butcher and her father was just rich. She is loyal and beautiful and funny and very "today" but her style is moneyed tradition. Although opulent and refined, almost everything in her house is dark. There are duck decoys everywhere. Preppy, moneyed people are into ducks. You're never allowed to throw anything away because it's been handed down from generation to generation. There's an antique bed that looks like a hot dog because it envelops whoever sleeps in it. *She* thinks it's her taste, but *I* think that she's so used to a certain kind of home that she's inherited that taste—it didn't develop to reflect her joyful spirit. That's just fine, though—people should surround themselves with what makes them happy.

I thought, for this chapter, it would be most helpful to give some ideas on how to best find and what to expect from a professional decorator, then to give you my own ideas on style and creativity in the home. From there you can proceed to break all the rules and do your own thing—or pick and choose from my and/or the professionals' suggestions. The hope is that you will be able to liberate your dreams of a wonderful home and find the confidence to take chances on color, furniture, and the total feel of your environment.

All About Decorators

WHY YOU MIGHT NEED ONE

• You don't know if you're baroque, modern, renaissance, or just plain unimaginative. In other words, a decorator would pull out that secret core of you that you know has style. And if there really *is* no core, a decorator could give you part of his or hers.

• You want to have a "total look," which will include breaking down walls, solving space and architectural problems, and you haven't a clue as to where to start or whom to hire to do it all.

• You need someone to do the dirty work of making *your* ideas reality: someone who knows the market, can transfer your taste to your home via the most terrific fabrics, prices, and selections. Mostly you don't have time to ferret out bargains, and you'd also like to be able to reach those "decorator only" show-rooms.

HOW DO I FIND A GOOD ONE?

Let's take "How do I find one?" first. We'll talk about "good" in a moment.

• Try looking in the home-decorating magazines for rooms you think are terrific and see who's credited for them.

• Try the model rooms of large department stores and ask to speak with the decorator responsible (Catch: If you use a store decorator, know that they're in business to push the store's merchandise, *first*. If you love the store, then it's fine. If not, stay away).

• Try the professional organizations to which decorators belong like the ASID (American Society of Interior Design) and ask for recommendations.

• Try your friends whose homes you love.

Now, let's get to the *good* decorator. Good is a relative term. I may love Jackson Pollock's paintings and you may think they're chicken dribbles. So check out recommended decorators by asking to see their work, their own houses, and their photographs of projects. If they tell you they won't show you anything because "each job is different" say goodbye: They're hiding something. Good, in other words, is what pleases you.

HOW MUCH SHOULD A DECORATOR COST?

Decorators usually earn their fees from taking a percentage of the amount of money you spend on furniture, contractors, and so on. Rarely does a decorator take a flat fee. Some charge by the hour, a risky practice if you're buying a decorator's services because top fees can vary from $75 to $150 an hour. I'd recommend not hiring a person who charges an hourly rate unless you're convinced that only he/she can do your home (you'd be wrong, of course).

To tell you the truth, sometimes you end up spending less if you use a decorator than you would by yourself, because decorators have sources unavailable to the buying public that may be very reasonable. And you do get the advantage of the decorator's expertise, flair, legwork, and stamina.

WHAT'S THE DANGER OF A DECORATOR?

A decorator's self-confidence may convince you that he or she knows what's better for you better than you do. A decorator doesn't. If you have the courage to experiment, do some research in magazines and decorating books, and don't mind pounding the pavements for buys and comparison shopping. I'm convinced you can create your own home scenario better than anyone else in the world. Because what's it all about? It's about *you*. Let's take it room by room and category by category.

The Kitchen

Most of all, the kitchen should be functional and do what it's supposed to do —help you and your family prepare creative, nourishing food. Since the kitchen, in many ways, is the heartbeat of a home, it should also be pretty with the colors and design that represent your idea of flair. My kitchen is a mixture of high tech —fashion follows function—and charm. A stove, for instance, should not be concerned with being avocado or lemon but with accommodating many pots. My stove is a huge black restaurant model that sounds ugly but, because of its size and potential, is absolutely fabulous. My fridge is also a restaurant model, big and see-through and made of unbreakable glass. Now *you* may not love a refrigerator whose contents are visible to the world, but you certainly ought to have a model that holds as much as possible, including space for *tall* bottles, rather than one that tells impeccable time and gives birth to ice cubes on the door.

Floors in kitchens make them unique. I've chosen hand-painted ceramic tiles, but you may favor earthy quarry tiles or a pristinely white vinyl . . . if you have a more sophisticated, monochromatic taste. Whatever you choose in color, a kitchen ought to be utilitarian with storage space galore provided in under-the-counter cabinets, hanging racks, over-the-counter shelves—all ideas that can be picked up in any home-decorating magazine. Walls can be used as "galleries" if you have space problems, with shelves that display cookbooks, herb gardens, spices, and other pleasing kitchen-y stock. Naturally you would not wish to display your cans of peas or stained pots—as I've seen in many kitchens. Every now and then, take a close look at what shows in your kitchen: Sometimes you get so used to seeing the bent and watermarked colander just hanging there that you don't realize how unappealing it is to a guest. Don't throw it out if it's serviceable —just get it out of sight! Some generalizations I've picked up from checking out some of the most chic kitchens in the world:

• Kitchen carpeting is never as easy to maintain as the manufacturers claim. There's always one spot, one frayed area that looks disgusting. I vote *no* to kitchen carpeting. It seems so dumb. And pretentious, anyway.

• *Corners* of kitchens are usually ignored. You can put a Lucite stepladder in a kitchen corner and use the steps for green or flowering plants, herb gardens, or cookbooks. Or, even in a tiny kitchen, build a little seat into a corner for someone to sit to keep you company or watch a pasta delight being created. A corner that's too small for a seat could house a rolling service cart with a Lucite or butcher-

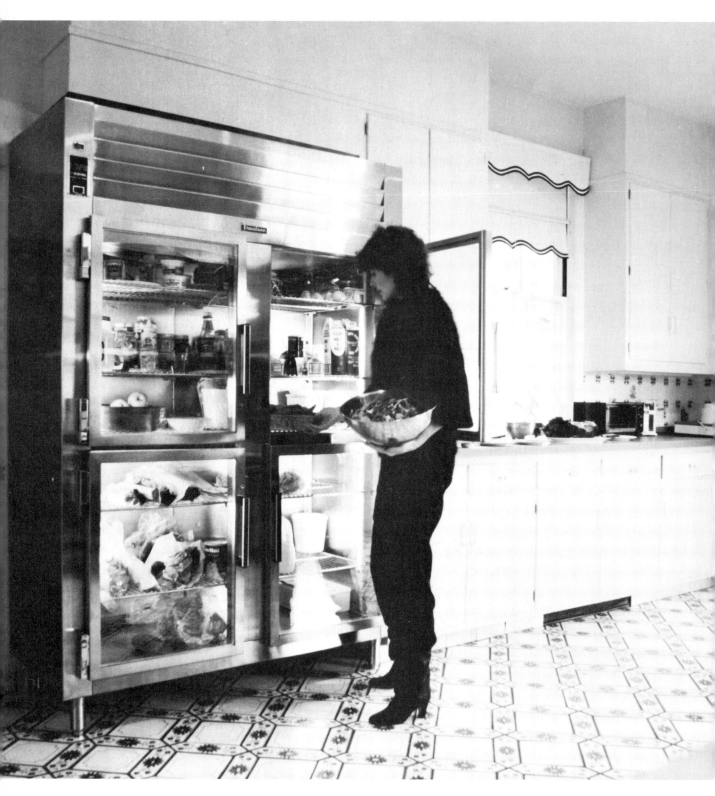

block top on which to prepare or store food, serve guests (you can always drape it with a gorgeous cloth to make it really elegant), or act as a rolling bar.

• Unless your garbage pail, rolling pins, spatulas, and other utensils are really gorgeous, don't display them. They collect dust and are horribly unappetizing. Build pegboard hanging places inside kitchen cabinet doors and closets, and hang everything away if possible. Hanging large, cumbersome items gets them out of the way and provides room for smaller items. Ditto for brooms, mops, and so on. They hang wonderfully if you screw a hook into the end of each long, wooden handle and another into the inside of a door or broom closet.

• I think that style in a kitchen consists of treating it as the room it is. That is, a kitchen can look like a kitchen and still be enormously attractive; it should not look like a boat, be as sterile as a hospital room, or as simply darling as a honeymoon cottage. A functional kitchen can be a joy to look at and still be recognizable as a kitchen. Above all, a kitchen should not have clutter. Clutter makes it an attic.

• Buy a cheap set of paints and play with them to determine the color for your kitchen. Try black-and-white geometrics, parrot greens, navy blues, bronzes —stunning, exciting combinations. Kitchens don't have to be yellow and white anymore—really. And include the ceiling in your decorating scheme, remembering that a light ceiling makes it look higher, and a darker tone will "lower" it.

Living and Dining Rooms, Not to Mention Dens

While it's surely easy to decorate these rooms when money is no object, the challenge is to do it within a budget and still do it smashingly.

I love seventeenth-century, hand-painted Japanese fabric on my walls, but I also love a hand-painted (by a friend or local artist) mural on a wall or ceiling to add an absolutely personal and unusual touch to a room. Prices can be negotiated on this.

Most of my crystal and linen come from auctions or advertised sellouts from estates. I look in the newspapers and pick up whole boxes of hand-appliquéd tablecloths from someone's grandmother. Sometimes you have to buy a whole "lot" with initialed napkins you can't use, for instance, just to get one truly magnificent item—but it always works out to be more economical, buying this way, than buying new. You can always use the initialed napkins as treasured and original gifts for someone whose name does start with a *Q*. My magnificent crystal was bought at auction at a fraction of the cost I'd have paid for it new.

Fabrics for upholstered furniture can be bought at wholesale outlets at a much reduced price because they might have tiny, invisible flaws. You *can* bring your own fabrics into many good department stores to be used on their furniture you intend to purchase. *Ask*—you have nothing to lose and the exquisite, unusual fabric you buy at discount prices can *make* a pedestrian piece of furniture look stunning.

Instead of wallpaper, fabrics make rooms inviting and you can buy them at outlets. A den with corduroy walls is warm and cozy.

You don't have to be born with a family fortune to have a richness of imagination. You just have to be born with daring. Try on this idea for openers. Imitating real marble or rare gems with cheap paste copies always looks offensive. You fool no one when you try to. But going all out, blatantly, wonderfully with an imitation that's *dramatically* false is fun and full of style: The French have been doing it for years and they call it *faux*. Having a mantelpiece painted in *faux* marble or a piece of furniture in *faux* tortoise by an experienced craftsperson makes a conversation piece with dash. As with everything else, too much *faux* is overkill and misses the point.

Details can warm up a room. My favorite piece in my living room is an absolutely magnificently huge red vase that dominates the whole room. I love red anyway: It reminds me that I'm here! Wonderful wood panels, unusual doorknobs, an extraordinary antique plate—all these are personal touches that spell your own style.

You're allowed to combine styles. That is, your room doesn't have to be exclusively Louis XVI or starkly Japanese. Eclecticism means combining elements from various sources, and that gives you freedom and added excitement.

My dining room chairs (and much of the other furniture in my house) were picked up for very little money at auctions. If the wood is fine, hand carved and elegant, I know I can always have it refinished and reupholstered for a fraction of the cost to buy new. So I do. And it's wonderful.

I believe in humor in my life and in my home. That means that friends know that if they want to give me a very special gift, it will be homemade and it will probably be an embroidered pillow. On an opulent sofa rests an exquisitely embroidered pillow that reads "Don't Talk to Me, I'm Having a Crisis." On a marble mantel sits a teeny pillow that says "Please Don't Sit on the Furniture." Touches of humor and wit enliven formality. They allow a guest to appreciate your home and also *love* it. I went to someone's house as a weekend guest once, and in the guest room was a magnificent, organdy, hand-painted pillow that read "You *are* going home Sunday, aren't you?" It made me laugh—and feel as if I didn't want to go home at all.

The Bathrooms

I love a knockout bathroom! My own bathroom is mostly utilitarian, a work space for my face, and thus is completely mirrored so when I have to make up, in any light, at any angle, a mirror is ready. But it's also beautiful with old art deco panels behind the tub and smoky mirrors around them. I love to paint the outside of tubs, which usually just *sit* in a room, unpretty and clumsy. Wallpaper creeping up the outside of a tub or a mural painted on it makes it an integral part of a room. Spray such work with fixatives to protect against dampness. The prettiest bathrooms I've seen have antique candelabras with real flickering candles when company comes, and touches of sterling silver, and china picture frames and stunning soaps: Bathrooms don't have to be pedestrian. Here's an idea I've often used to bring true elegance to this room: I have a local carpenter construct a vanity around an old-fashioned sink from the cheapest wood he can find. The newspaper often lists sellouts of builders' overpurchases, and one can buy sheets of old Mexican onyx, real marble, or stunning slate at truly rock-bottom prices, which the carpenter can then affix to the wood, and you have a magnificent vanity for very little money. Try buying an onyx vanity at one of the multitudes of fancy bathroom shops that proliferate in big cities—they're prohibitively expensive! And if you save up the carpentry you want done, you'll probably get lower prices from a craftsperson who appreciates the greater volume of work.

In my own upstairs bathroom, which is a wonderfully large room, I've thrown a colorful hand-hooked rug over the tiles and hung family pictures I love. Over all, my favorite Portuguese-china ceramic cat watches impassively.

Bedrooms

Bedrooms are retreats, trysting places, and fantasy islands as far as I'm concerned. They're the most personal place in the home and they should be inviting as heck. You can recreate in your bedroom the pages of a magazine, the colors of the whole outside, or the wonder of a special trip you've taken if you open your mind to the unusual. Bedrooms should really tell the story of the people who live there—with the grandest style of all. Art, colors, and personal possessions say "Zachary lives here" (if he does). For example, Zachary's bedroom in our city apartment has walls that are papered in giant Z's. In his country bedroom, the wallpaper is of his own choosing—sailing ships that he loves and an old army bed that we resurrected from a thrift shop and painted. Over the bed is a sign that says "PRESENTING DELOREAN." On another wall is a painting I've done of him sleeping with dream images of baseball games, swimming holes, unicorns floating airily about his sleeping self.

One of my favorite additions to a bedroom is fresh flowers, and when I can't have them fresh, because of the season, I have them in porcelain.

A great luxury in a bedroom is a plush coverlet, and my friends have paid small fortunes for their down comforters. If one were to go to a wholesale stuffing place (this one did) and buy down stuffing by the pound, go to an outlet fabric place to pick up some magnificent "second" in fabric, and then go to the Yellow

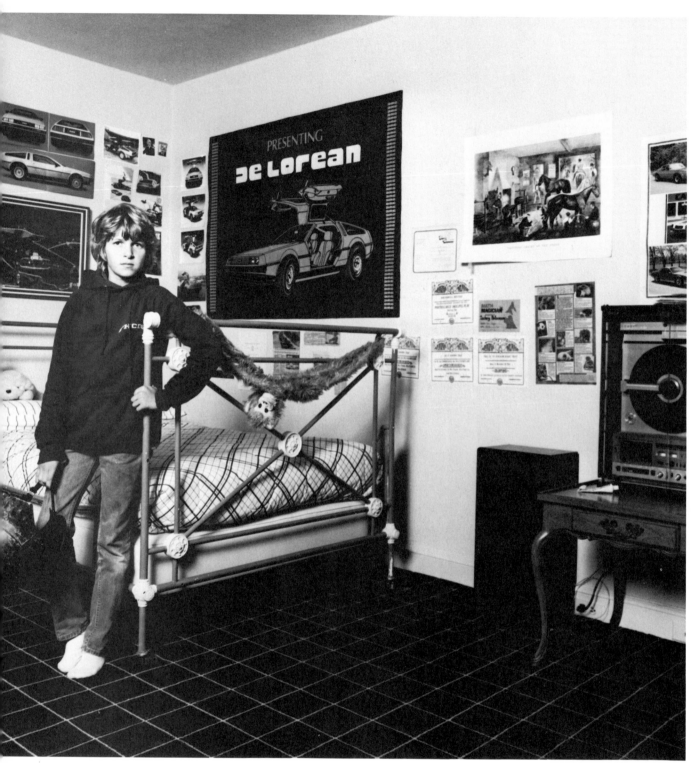

Presenting—Zachary DeLorean

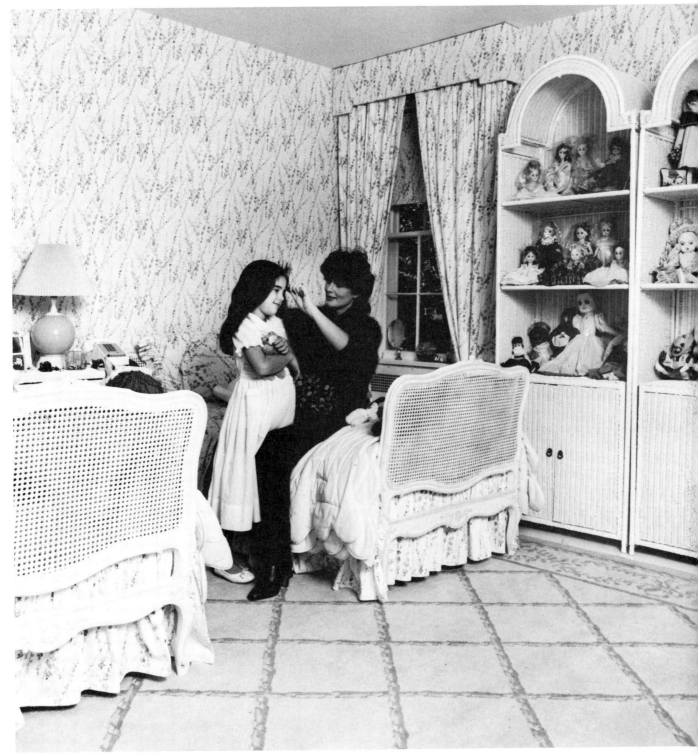

Kathryn's wickery garden bedroom

Pages to find a local seamstress, one could have such a plush comforter made for about two hundred dollars as opposed to the thousand it will cost your cousin Cynthia, who only knows from shopping in department stores.

The same local dressmaker who makes the comforter can make drapes, furniture covers, and bedspreads from your material at far less than retail prices. The local dressmaker, incidentally, is a *wonderful* woman to get to know. She can, if she's talented, and if your payments are fair, save you money and bring hand-tailored elegance to your whole home.

You can use the colors of nature in your bedroom much as you use them in clothing. A "seascape" bedroom could have the beige and white of shells and the blue of the sky and the sea; a garden room could have the verdant greens of the grasses and the exuberantly delicate wildflower colors on pillows, spreads, and carpeting . . . with a white wicker fence translated into wicker furniture. If you're into simplicity, the serenity and purity of tatami mats, shoji screens, and rattan brings Japan to mind. And never be afraid to throw an element of romance or nostalgia in a bedroom that is not predominantly ruffles and chintz: surprise makes for delight in decorating—especially in a bedroom.

My own bedroom is covered with green, pink, and white flowers. I bought our headboard at auction for under a hundred dollars and had it recovered in the same fabric that brings our walls to life. The two night tables were also auction bargains, which I grabbed at fifty dollars each: They were a dark and undistinguished wood, stained with the weight of years when I saw them, but now they're green and white and cheerful after a couple of hours with my paintbrush. I had an overhead cornice built from the cheapest wood and, when covered in the bed and wall fabric, it makes a fairy-tale canopy for my bed.

Closets

Too many people ignore closets. Looking into the same dark recess every day can be downright depressing. Take linen closets, for example. You can apply lacy, pink ribbons along shelf edges, line walls with old but still pretty sheets, stash tiny bags of dried herbs or potpourri on shelves to make the whole closet smell sweet. I've papered John's closet with a paper that says "I Love You" in white on chocolate a million times and every time he opens the door, he tells me, he feels a glow of warmth. Old wooden bars in closets can be transformed with adhesive-backed plastic that comes in many colors and snaps on in a second to allow your clothes on their hangers to smoothly glide along the bar. Glazed chintz cotton on the walls, a mural painted on a door, a Flokati rug on the floor—closets *can* have style!

Guest Rooms

Guest rooms don't have to be enormous to look terrific and be comfortable. You can cover a wall with fabric or grass cloth, a bed with a wonderful antique quilt, and a floor with straw-colored sisal matting. A rocking chair is lovely in a guest room as is adequate lighting. If you put old furniture or attic junk in a guest room, make sure it's freshly painted so as to look charming instead of rusty. Fresh flowers, extra blankets and sheets, a small radio or TV, a clock, ashtrays for smokers, and books are all wonderful to add to the guest room. I always make sure a guest bathroom is stocked with:

- Fresh toothbrushes, mouthwash, toothpaste, razor and blades;
- Sample bottles of shampoo and conditioner;
- Fresh soap—*always* fresh soap. Even a *little*-used soap is gauche;
- Four or five little tampons wrapped with a pretty ribbon;
- A little bottle of Pepto-Bismol in case, God forbid, my cooking talks back;
- Aspirin;
- Clean towels—not that fancy, unusable guest-towel sort, but big, plush absorbent ones;
- A magazine rack with bathroom reading is always thoughtful.

From the Specific to the General

It's difficult to be terribly specific in terms of decorating style because each person is so uniquely special, but there are some sound and general rules I've learned that make decorating a home a breeze. For example:

CROSS THE COLOR LINE

Sometimes you have to break the rules when it comes to color. You're allowed to have raspberry walls instead of white ones. You're allowed to throw a patchwork quilt on your bed instead of a traditional monochromatic bedspread. Pick up the threads in an antique rug and let them be your guide for color in that room. Or look into your *closet* for ideas. We tend to dress in the colors that flatter us and we've usually given more thought to our clothes than to our surroundings; therefore, assume that the colors that look good on you, and please you, will also be wonderful in your home. A color that gives a psychological lift on your back will do the same in your living room.

Remember: Warm colors like reds, oranges, and yellows on a wall can make a room look smaller, but red used on a couch or chair can make the furniture look larger. Cool colors like blues, beige, violets on a wall can make the room look larger. Break up the cool colors with some warm fabrics and sunny stuff.

FABRICS AND STUFFINGS

Pillows and chair seats lend coziness and warmth to a room, but the Dacron and foam you find in most ready-made furniture is hard and lumpy. Hie thee down to a stuffing store and buy 100 percent *down* cheaply, and have your furniture pillows and covering custom-made, if possible (supplying your own fabric from wholesale houses is sometimes even cheaper than buying a piece ready-made—and it's infinitely nicer and more personal). Many department stores are willing to make furniture with your own choice of fabric and stuffing, and again, don't forget the local seamstress who can transform an old couch with new slip-covers. A quick guide to fabric: One hundred percent natural products like wool, linen, silk, and heavy cotton *breathe* and are longer lasting than synthetics—no matter what the salesperson tells you. The worst things you can use in your home are plastic-type fabrics to which you stick and which invariably make embarrassing sounds as you plop down on them.

"Soil-resistant" fabrics aren't.

Fabric should be appealing in a tactile way. One should want to run a finger over inviting velvet, shiny chintz, lush corduroy. If it feels cheap, it probably is—and will last about five and a half minutes.

A WORD ABOUT LEATHER: It's lovely when it's the real top-grain material (look for sales), but it's worse than terrible when it's imitation. A synthetic vinyl does not give an aura of style, and it cracks, gets hot and is miserable to sit on and often has a funny smell. Glove leather and suede are soft and silky but wear poorly. Never use furniture polish, ammonia, oil, or Ajax-type abrasives to clean leather. Just dust and wipe clean with lukewarm water and a mild soap, then rinse and dry. Don't overload on leather if you want to avoid an "office" look to your home.

HERE'S A TIP: Many beautiful fabrics today are blends, and the manufacturers claim that the blend of a natural and synthetic fabric lends for hardy, durable material. Not true. I have it on very good authority and even better experience that a material is only as strong as the weakest threads, and that means if you buy a couch that's half silk and half rayon, the fabric will last only as long as it would if it were all rayon. If you like the blend for its appearance, fine, but don't buy a blend thinking it's stronger than an all natural weave.

ANOTHER TIP ABOUT FABRICS: Detached pillows are always a greater buy than backs and seats that are part of the couch or chair construction: You can turn them over to spread the attrition of use every now and then and clean them far more easily.

WINDOWS

They're our ticket to the world. They ought not, I think, be smothered in heavy, never-let-the-light-in drapes. Unless the world outside your window is a brick wall, make the window frame a picture frame that encircles the landscape outside (and the landscape can be green trees or bustling city—each is wonderful in its own way). If your landscape is a brick wall, reconsider the drapes—in a light fabric. Here are some suggestions for decorating windows:

• Consider a window seat, built from plywood and covered with tiles or pillows, to curl up and read on, to put plants on, to add the most inviting seating in the room.

• Consider a simple shade made from the fabric of your couch or chairs to pull the room together.

• Consider crisp louvers or vertical blinds in bamboo, wood, woven yarn, or aluminum.

• Consider fresh, airy curtains—billowy, sheer, embroidered.

• *Do not* consider heavy, curvy, curly, thick draperies, which are dated and dust collectors.

• Last, consider a Japanese shoji screen treatment: nonopaque, exquisitely simple doors on a track that create a sense of tranquility and can be closed for privacy and opened to let in the outdoors.

THE BACKDROPS

Think of walls and ceilings as giant canvases. Their decoration or covering can be as exciting as any furniture and art objects within the room. You can cover your walls with cloth, paper, paint, or wood. You can cover them with tapestry, rugs, shelves, or books. You can paint a trompe l'oeil (trick of the eye) design that makes you think a green woods, a window, or a vase of flowers is where it isn't. You can have a mural on the ceiling or on just one wall. Wall and ceiling coverings can make a room live, provide a backdrop for your "things," cozy up the place, and make people gasp with delight when they enter. Study the magazines and the model rooms in department stores for ideas.

THE IMPLEMENTS

Everything that's within those walls and under that ceiling is an implement. It carries out an effect or a function. Don't make the implements *permanent* is the best advice I can give you. Change your surroundings. Never be "finished" with your home. Change your dishes, your throw pillows, your plant holders, your bedspread, your furniture coverings from time to time—not all of them all the time, but one or two small changes in your environment every so often gives you a new lease on life. Just as minds stagnate, homes can also if they don't move with your whims and personality growth. Accessories, books, and everything in your home ought to be *friendly* (stunning and chic *can* be friendly).

ILLUSIONS

Just as makeup gives an illusion of beauty, mirrors can give an illusion of space. Mirroring a bar or a bathroom totally opens it up and gives it drama.

Mirrors fill unused and "dead" space, create "set apart" areas, even change shapes.

A ROOM OF ONE'S OWN

Virginia Woolf wrote that every woman needed her own space—even if it was closet sized. You can share vacations, money, and children, dinners, beds, and bathrooms—but in the end, you need a quiet place of your own to withdraw to from the world for a while. Think about converting a closet, a small hall, a section of the bedroom that can be screened off for your use alone. I use the room of my own as a tonic and a pick-me-up every single day.

A MENTOR OF ONE'S OWN

In this case, it's the magazines that are the teachers and sources of inspiration. Now never make the mistake of thinking that those *House Beautiful* rooms are easy to replicate. They look stunning, and they took informed, studied, and sophisticated effort to create them; however, it's not the *whole* room you're after. It's an idea, an imagination jogger, a jumping-off point. A room that's being touted for its eclectic furniture may attract your attention just because of the good-looking ceiling graphic it portrays—not for the furniture at all. You show the graphic to a painter (maybe it's a simple stripe that encircles a room but makes the difference between smart and dull) and you're in business.

Going, Going, Gone!

I love to find the treasure in the junk trove. Here are some thoughts about auctions:

1. There's two kind of auctions: The high-class gallery type and the country auction. Both are great. An auction is a show, a happening, a theater piece. Also you can buy good things. Don't be intimidated or spurred on by either the cool or frantic behavior of others. You may end up buying something you don't want, need, or like.

2. Be open-minded. You can't shop at an auction with a specific item in mind—you may wait for it forever. Instead, check out what's available. You may find a treasure to transform your kitchen when you have your mind on your den.

3. Think creative! What one person has thrown out—say, a funky side chair, may be funky in its original state but transformed with paint and new fabric it can become fabulous.

4. If it's an outside country auction and the weather's not terrific—that's

your best bet for a good price. A small crowd means a reasonable bidding level. If it's summertime at Parke-Bernet and the beautiful people are all at the Hamptons, go to the auction. But if the weather's lousy, and everyone's in town, stay home from the auction.

Six Decorating Secrets I've Learned

1. ALL THAT GLITTERS IS NOT GOLD. Just because it's gilded with a famous or recognizable name doesn't mean it's pure gold. Tiffany turned out some oinkers. So did Chippendale. So did Picasso. If *you* don't love it, don't hang it.

2. CAN YOU LIVE WITH IT? Before you decide on any bedroom wallpaper, ask yourself this question: Could I be locked in this room for three days and look at these walls without screaming?

3. NEVER BUY ANYTHING that makes you say, "Isn't that the most *precious* thing?" You will soon grow to despise it.

4. TAKE CHANCES. You can always recover the Dreadful Orange Mistake. If you always play it safe, you'll have a boring home.

5. SOMEONE ONCE SAID, "Never buy anything that's flamboyant, freaky, or gimmicky." I disagree. *One* flamboyant, freaky, or gimmicky thing in a room can illustrate passion, humor, or strength. Two or more f.f.g. things can illustrate lack of style.

6. MUDDY COLORS ARE NEVER MAGICAL. Neither is an abundance of ducks.

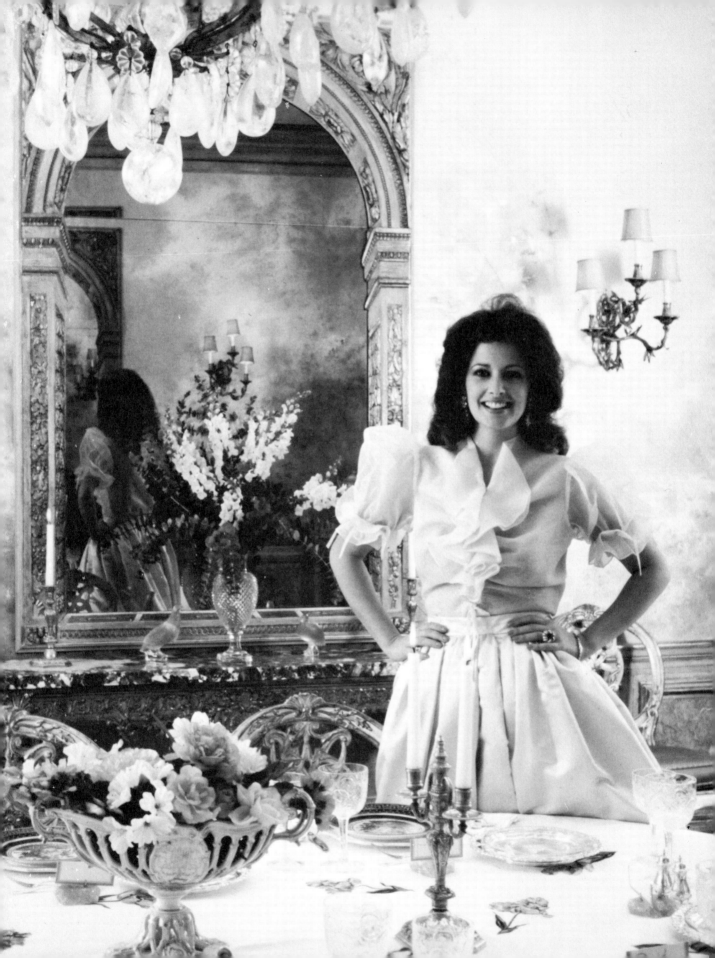

Chapter 8

PARTY STYLE

I LOVE to entertain.

I love to give big parties and I love to give small parties. I love to cook and to feed my friends. And, I say this without very much modesty, I love being the central object in my own setting.

Obviously it's easier to entertain when money is no object. I've made dinner parties that have set me back thousands of dollars—not counting the flowers. I've also been to homes where I've been entertained in the kind of style that a fortune of money can inspire—I'm talking butlers, champagne, caviar and homes that turn into tropical fantasies by the time a fancy florist and a big check make friends. Sure, that's style. Style in the grand fashion.

But style in the real world demands just as much elegance and even more creativity minus the big bucks. I knew it in my early years when my mother entertained lavishly and deliciously on very little; I knew it in the early days of my career when I did the same; and now I'm learning it all over again.

Just as dressing with style means attention to details, so does entertaining. You can have Vanderbilt wealth and silver inherited from Henry VIII and your dinner party will still be a disaster if it doesn't have *heart*. Heart doesn't imply butlers waiting on you. A buffet can be as glamorous and stylish as a formal sit-down dinner. But heart does mean a gift of relaxation, entertainment (not jugglers —just good conversation), and good food that you offer to your guests. The first thing you ought to consider when planning a party is the guest list . . . that's the heart of the heart.

The Guest List for a Perfect Party

You'll need, first of all, someone who values language. Since snappy conversation is the key ingredient to almost any kind of party, a guest who knows how to make original—even controversial—conversation is always a plus. I feel enlivened leaving a party where I've been in a verbal sparring meet as opposed to leaving a party bored to tears by polite and innocuous word exchanges. You can't invite too many of these controversial types because they tend to clash. One is terrific—three are a pain in the neck.

You'll need your "entertainer." Oh, not Joan Rivers or Buddy Hackett (although if you can get *them—terrific!*) but the pal who always makes everyone giggle because he or she tells a great story or has a wry way of looking at things. Avoid joke tellers. They put a wet blanket on festivities. No one likes holding still for interminable minutes listening to convoluted jokes where the punch line is *never* worth the wait.

Ignore the pompous manuals that tell you to invite only people with disparate interests and occupations. I've found that people with the same interests and even the same occupations don't make for dull but for excited and exciting guests; each always has a better story to top the others and they all understand what the others are talking about. Obviously, there are no firm and hard rules except maybe you'd always want to avoid an all-accountants party. All lawyers, all entertainers, all brain surgeons, and all journalists parties have been known to be delightful.

Never pair people off—either at the table or in any designated groups. It's offensive and silly to be told you *must* sit near a man if you're a woman or talk to a producer if you're a starlet. Style consists of assuming the intelligence and ability of your guests to discover the other guests who will most turn them on.

Never invite so many guests that *you* can't be there for each of them; it is not stylish to throw a barn warming, I feel, where the barn is the center of attraction. A person of style is very much a part of the conversation, the mood, and the momentum of her own party—she's not there just to serve and offer a meeting ground for others.

If there's a "crowd" that always hangs out together, it's not a terrific idea to invite only them—no matter how congenial they are—to a party. New faces among the old lend a certain zest to a group.

I've often read that you shouldn't invite too many "superstars" to the same party—because each requires undivided attention. Nonsense. Superstars, whether they be famous trial lawyers, movie stars, musicians, politicians, or moneymakers are usually aggressive, stimulating questioners *and* answerers; the very fact of their being powerhouses makes for a powerhouse party, with each trying to be his or her most endearing best. Never be afraid of strong people—they make for a stimulating atmosphere.

Essayist Quentin Crisp once said, "It's not true that stylists surround themselves with dullards. Conversation stimulates conversation; wit provokes wit. Every hostess knows no party can be called a success until everyone is talking and no one is listening."

Finally, if the purpose of your party is to "pay back"—the reciprocation of social obligation—don't invite me. It's got to be a bomb.

Dinner Logistics

Okay, you know whom you'll invite, you've set the date and the menu—what next? *Write it down!* Get a small notebook and jot down a list of things you'll need to buy, store by store. For example:

Fish Store	*Grocery Store*
Clams	Pasta
Shrimps	Lettuce
	Etc.

I guarantee you if you don't write it down, you'll forget it!

THE DAY BEFORE THE PARTY

- Do all shopping, if possible. It makes for a far less harried hostess.
- If you can, cook whatever is possible to prepare in advance.
- Polish the silver.
- Set the table.
- Get out the linens you'll use, vases for flowers, make extra ice cubes.

THE DAY OF THE PARTY

- Buy and arrange the flowers.
- Set out pretty towels, candles, and flowers in the bathrooms.
- Prepare the remainder of the food and store in fridge, if necessary.

Now for the Specifics

THE SHOPPING

It's always advisable to shop where the proprietor knows you and to involve him or her in your dinner party. Describe the menu—ask for advice. Make friends with your grocer. I don't say it's necessary to invite him (or her) for dinner, but be cordial and interested in his family and work.

Sounds simplistic, but it works. If someone cares about you, he'll slap your hands off the wilted lettuce and go in the back to pick the freshest of the fresh for you. Making friends with the butcher, the greengrocer, the florist is the smartest thing a consumer can do. Instead of treating a grocer as the keeper of the tomatoes—try finding out about his wife, his life. Try sharing yours a bit. It will pay off in the best cuts of meat and the finest produce—as well as a pleasant relationship. Naturally you won't involve the checkout person in a huge super-market with your problems, but even the huge supermarket has a *person* in charge of the meat, a *person* in charge of the produce—and always the same person. Make him your ally and friend.

THE FLOWERS

To me flowers make a party. They can cost a small fortune, as everyone knows, but if you use your smarts, you'll find the wholesale flower market (find out where your florist buys his or *her* flowers) and shop there. Go at a time when it's not busy (early in the morning is the worst: No one will pay you one bit of attention), and plan to buy more than a bunch of daisies. Still, you can pick carefully; you can even bring along the containers you wish to use and ask for suggestions. There's no question that fifty dollars' worth of flowers can be bought for less than half that price—and sometimes a quarter of the price. If there is no wholesale flower market nearby, call around to find the best retail prices. And don't go for the usual single "arrangement" in the center of the table. Sometimes an individual flower at each place setting, or just one or two stunning and exotic flowers off-center on a table can make your party really exquisite and different. There's nothing more boring than the predictable centerpiece of carnations, roses and ferns. The flowers for my party—all of them that you see pictured—cost under twenty dollars . . . and that includes some flowers in the bathroom, not pictured. Think vivid colors for flowers. Think spring flowers in the wintertime. Think anemones, tulips, irises, freesia, rubrum lilies. Think baby's breath to sprinkle here and there. Do not think pallid pink.

Think about containers for flowers by casting an appraising eye on the container-type objects in your house. There's no law that says flowers must go in a vase. If you take a low glass jar, fill it with black rocks and one or two blue irises, you have a Japanese sculpture for your table. "Frogs," those little, green, many-spiked objects that can be placed in containers and hidden by ferns, are wonder-

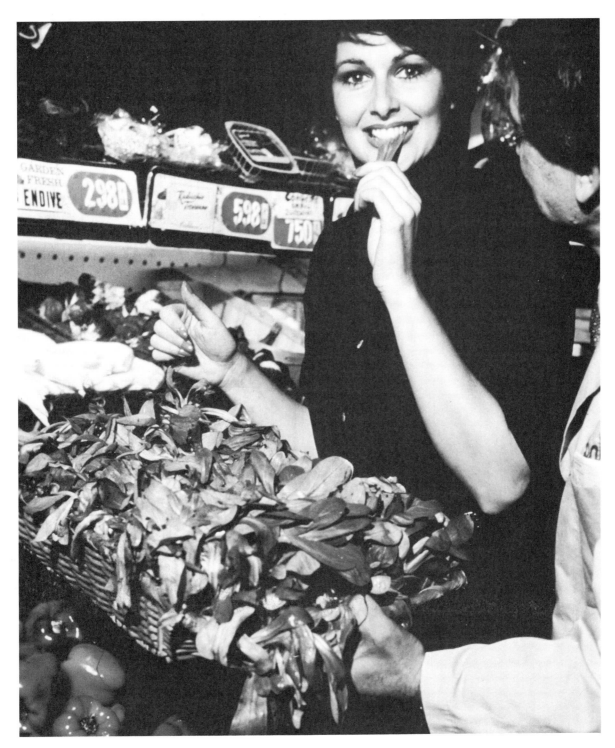

*Sampling the produce at Balducci's
market the day before the Sixty-Dollar
Formal Dinner for Twelve*

ful for flower arrangements as is "oasis," the stuff that looks like green Styrofoam into which, when soaked, you can stick stems. An addition of a product like Floral Life (obtainable from any florist), or about a tablespoon of something sweet, like 7-Up, or a tablespoon of Clorox bleach to a quart of water makes flowers last longer. Cut each stem on an angle before placing the flower in water, and if you want to ensure really long life, cut each stem a little bit every day. Misting flowers with fine sprays keeps them fresh longer than just watering them from the stem.

If you have a flat simple arrangement—flowers in a wide, low-sided dish, there's nothing prettier than some petals floating around it. Check out the colors on your container, by the way—when you can pick up the same color in one or two of the flowers, it's pretty.

A LITTLE FIRST AID FOR FLOWERS: Wilting tulips? Let them sit with their stems in cold water and ice cubes for a few hours—a miraculous revival will occur! Ditto with violets.

Wilting heather? Split the stems and place them in hot water to revive.

How to keep certain frail species vital?
- *Roses:* The water in container should be only a third the length of stem;
- *Zinnias, marigolds:* Remove buds or leaves that would be under water;
- *Lilies:* Remove the stamen;
- *Gladioli:* Put five tablespoons of vinegar mixed in a quart of water in the container.

DRESSING THE TABLE

Dishes and glasses count as much as food. Put the culinary masterpiece of a four-star chef on a cracked and suspiciously yellowing plate and it's almost inedible. I love pretty dishes, and mine are expensive, but if I didn't have the money to buy exquisite china, I'd still have appealing plates. Every community has a store that sells clear, simple crystal or glass plates. Wineglasses should be of perfect lucidity—even though they're not Baccarat crystal. You can obtain ceramic china of marvelous color and inexpensive origin. Whatever you do— don't use dishes that imitate: brassy, gold paint on dishes trying to be Limoges china makes them look like shooting gallery prizes. The best is always the simplest and the truest to form. Clear glass and Lucite can be gorgeous. Style is not made of crystal and bone china—it's made from flair and honesty. Still, if you won't be satisfied with anything but the finest dishes and glasses, do what I do and shop the auctions, the antique stores, and the estate close outs, where you can pick up china and crystal, not dirt cheaply, but at a far better price than if you'd gone into a retail store.

Here's another possibility: Look around for a friend who's traveling abroad or to one of the islands. Very often china and crystal indigenous to the area are far less expensive bought there and shipped home. Waterford crystal, for instance, costs almost half as much in Dublin (counting the shipping) as it does in New York.

Once the food is on whatever dishes you use, whether it's to be served buffet style or formally, each plate ought to be an art form. A plate of yellow saffron rice is enhanced with sprinkles of green parsley. Melon can be scooped out in balls, served with mint sprigs. A scoop of ice cream served in a hollow chocolate form with a fresh flower on the plate is elegant; a plate of just ice cream is pedestrian, styleless. A meat loaf, looked at with vision, can be an aesthetic experience.

SETTING THE TABLE

I've been to dinner parties where the food was mediocre, the hostess was clumsy, but the table was set so magnificently, almost all else was forgiven! I've always felt that those who care about food ought to make the serving of it an experience, a *presentation*. Eating should never be casual—it should be an event . . . even when you're eating all by yourself. Too many diets are sabotaged because we tend to stuff food unceremoniously down our faces; if we made it a ceremony of sorts, a careful appreciation of the food—we'd eat less and enjoy it more. I think of my table as a painting—and a unique one at that, with the plates, flowers, cloths, and food as pleasing to the eye as the meal should be to the palate. Here are some suggestions:

• At each place, wrap the silverware in a pretty napkin and tie it up with a ribbon bow to complement the flowers on the table. You might even place a flower in each bow.

• Individual place cards for each person can be written in fancy lettering on a plain card and inserted in a tiny porcelain rose, or a Lucite holder. Such place card holders are available in every gift store and, of course, can be used over and over; it's a nice way to tell people where you want them to sit and it personalizes your party.

• Candles on the table are romantic and set a mood, but they should never be scented candles. Pasta or roast beef smelling like gardenia incense kind of takes the edge off the appetite.

• Flowers can be sprinkled in tiny, individual containers all over the table, at each place setting, or in the center.

• Put the season or the occasion on your table. If it's Christmas, pine cones spread around the table are pretty. Or tiny red-and-green ornaments in the center of the table. Or holly. If it's Halloween, a pumpkin, used as a container for your flower arrangement (but, please, not your ordinary, smiling, toothy jack-o'-lantern!). A *classy* pumpkin with a different expression, perhaps a bow tie or earrings or something else amusing. Chocolate eggs have adorned my table at a party near Easter. An engagement party might feature a papier-mâché diamond ring nestled in the flowers.

• Consider a centerpiece of vegetables or fruit. A huge bowl of the reddest, roundest apples makes a dynamite center—especially if you set miniature "love apples" in front of each plate and tack a name card on each one. The arrangement of great green stalks of asparagus lining a circular bowl with piles of purple grapes in their center looks like a painting. Purple-black eggplants, sun-orange bell peppers—use your imagination!

Small Talk

Don't knock it. Small talk is a social grace that's essential, and when polished to perfection it breaks down barriers and opens strangers up to each other in a delightful way. As dogs sniff each other to decide what their relationship will be, people do their sniffing through the "Hello, how are you, what's new, I like your bracelet" routine. Good small talkers make a party terrific, and if it doesn't happen naturally, it's up to the hostess to get things moving.

One way of doing that is through introductions. It would be good if people wore labels with terse information about themselves—"Rich Bigot"; "Suzie Feminist"; "John Radio Announcer." Because they don't, the hostess has to supply the labels by way of introduction. "This is Joe who just did that article about palimony—and this is Susan who teaches Chinese cooking," and they're off and running about palimony and ginger root. If *you* are the guest, small talk depends in part on your doing your homework before the party. "So, you're the guy I hear makes the greatest chocolate mousse in town?" or "I understand you're from Paris."

Read the paper before you have a party. If no one brings up the article about cloning, when there's a lull in the conversation, think of a way to get it in . . . and that will spark the small talk. Or ask someone what his political opinion on a certain issue is. Or ask someone what her first job was—everyone remembers that and loves to talk about it.

Some people use flattering bluntness:
- I saw you across the room and wanted to tell you you have the nicest smile here.
- I just felt I wanted to talk with you.

You questions are sure-fire small talk openers:
- How do *you* feel about the work you do?
- How do *you* think I should open this bottle of wine?
- I'm doing a survey for a magazine piece: Can *you* tell me the best restaurant in this town?

At a party, try to avoid giving endless details about operations, dogs, or children; avoid telling intimate things about yourself—that makes people feel awkward; avoid picking things off people's collars (lint, hairs, and so on). And don't ask professional people for free advice—nothing kills a conversation faster.

Most of all, at your own party, be energetic, be warm as you small talk: That is absolutely infectious!

What happens when you are involved in chitchat at a party and simply must move on into the kitchen to check the soufflé? Extract yourself gracefully by bringing someone else into the picture: "Doug, come over here and listen to this hilarious stuff Jim's been telling me." And then, "Excuse me you two—I have to check the stove."

Finally, make your guests feel comfortable in conversation by paying attention, looking into their eyes, responding. Someone once said, "No one would listen to anyone else speak if he didn't know it was his turn next." Well, your turn is coming: Hear your guests out.

Seating

I think the tradition of separating couples at dinner parties is foolish. I always like to know that the person I'm most comfortable with is on one side—in case things get boring or tense. One can always talk to the people across the table or on the other side. I suppose if I were having a dinner party where I knew that three of the four couples invited despised each other, I'd separate them, but otherwise I think enforced separation is silly. If you notice, at most parties where seating is not designated, couples always seem to sit together; that's because it's comfortable and natural that way. There are plenty of opportunities to talk to others even when your spouse is alongside. When we're invited out and placed at different tables, John always changes the place cards when the hostess isn't looking. Naturally that mortifies me, but I'm always relieved to have him on one side. I can always think of things to bother *him* with if my other partner is dull.

If you're having a casual buffet, stack tables are great, but never hesitate to ask your guests to pull up the floor—even in black tie—if you don't have enough table room. I've generally found that as soon as one lowers herself under the seat level, the inhibition level starts to drop . . . and that makes for zippier conversation.

Help!

You may be able to do it all yourself, and if you can (and I often do) more power to you. Still, there may come that special party where you'll want to hire some outside assistance to make a smoother and easier evening for you. Here are some suggestions about that. First of all, you will probably want to know:

- Where do I find such a person?
- How much will it cost me?
- What are the responsibilities of hired help?

WHERE DO I FIND SUCH A PERSON?

The first thing I do is call my friends and ask if they have any specific recommendations. If they have no bright ideas, I consult the phone book and call some local catering services who generally have lists of free-lance maids and bartenders. You might check the employment agencies listed in the phone book, but when going through this source make very sure that the agency is certified and bonded (insured for any losses you may incur from dishonest help helping themselves to your silverware). You should also consider the teenage children of friends who will not take unkindly to putting on a clean dress or suit for the evening in order to earn a few extra dollars. Also, check into the local high schools or colleges to see if they have student placement bureaus. Finally, professional organizations of actors, writers, police, and so on often have lists of members who "moonlight" to pick up some extra cash when they're not working at their professions. Again, make sure that these organizations have some means of "bonding" the people they send out to you. Newspapers and professional journals usually list numbers to call for such moonlighters.

HOW MUCH WILL IT COST ME?

Anywhere from twenty dollars an evening for a friend's son or daughter to the minimum rate charged by a professional organization (at least five dollars an hour). Whether you pay by the hour or by the evening, make sure the rate is set in advance with whomever you hire so there are no misunderstandings. If you don't pay a helper through an agency, pay is expected right after the party: Almost no one is thrilled to have to submit a bill and have you attend to paying it when you take care of your other monthly expenses. Tip? Sure, if you've been very happy with the service.

WHAT ARE THE RESPONSIBILITIES OF HIRED HELP?

Decide and clearly explain each person's responsibilities an hour or so before the party begins. Here are some ideas:

A BARTENDER: The role of a bartender is to mix drinks (he's [or she's] not responsible for exotic fancies—anyone who asks for a banana daiquiri should get a polite explanation that it's not available), clean glasses, clean out ashtrays periodically, and straighten out the "cocktails room" when the guests go into dinner so they can come back to a clean room after dinner. He or she should be asked to set up the bar with ice cubes, mixes, liquor, limes—whatever is needed.

A WAITRESS OR WAITER: Unless you hire a consummate professional, sit down a day or at least an hour or so before the dinner and play Make-Believe Dinner, where the hired person is the guest and you play the waitress. Then serve each course (simulated, of course, with just the dishes and not the food) as you wish it served. Some basic rules:
  • Food is served to the *left* of the guest and plates are removed from the *right* of the guest.

• Wine and water are served to the *right* of the guest, where the glasses are placed at the place setting.

• Dishes are *never* scraped and stacked when clearing the table, à la luncheonette style. The helper may clear the table taking a plate in each hand and never using a tray, either. (At really, really posh dinners, only one plate at a time is removed from the table: It's terribly boring.)

• For a variation in serving one plate at a time: The host may carve the meat or fowl, the helper waits at his side and then takes the plate of meat to each guest. Vegetables can be placed in large serving bowls on the table (one for each side) from which the guests serve themselves.

• The host may quite properly get up and refill wineglasses.

Before the party, make sure you've "walked" your helper through your kitchen so she (or he) knows where to place the dishes and silverware after she's finished washing them.

A COOK: If you prefer not to do the cooking yourself, hire an *experienced* cook. Discuss the menu with her (or him), in advance, ask her to tell you how much preparation time she'll need, and make sure she will do the dishes.

Glittering Generalities

WINE: Don't be iron-bound to the "white wine with fish and chicken, red wine with meat" rule. That's pompous. Serve what you like, but make sure the white wine is chilled and the red is at room temperature.

TIP: If you rub the round rim of an open wine bottle with a sheet of waxed paper, it won't drip.

TIP: If the recipe calls for wine as an ingredient, *never* buy "cooking wine" in the supermarket—it's always awful. For just about the same price you can buy a "real" bottle of wine, which is infinitely better.

TIP: Dry vermouth can always be substituted for white wine.

NEVER COOK VEGETABLES TO A DRY, DRAB DEATH. The very essence, the true state, of vegetables emerges when you steam them for just a few minutes to a brilliant green or rich yellow.

PASTA is the most satisfying dish in the world, and you can dress it up with bright basil leaves, clam sauce, vegetables, meats, parsley . . .

PREPARE SALADS IN ADVANCE. Lettuce can keep crisp if rinsed and wrapped in clean Turkish towels and then refrigerated. Avocado can be kept bright by sprinkling a little lemon juice on it or putting the avocado seed in the salad bowl until ready to serve.

UNMOLD MOLDS IN ADVANCE to avoid last-minute hysteria: Use warm water and allow them to reharden in the refrigerator if they are a little melted out.

WHIPPED CREAM CAN ALSO BE PREPARED IN ADVANCE. Either refrigerate it if it's just a matter of keeping it intact for a couple of hours, or freeze it in individual mounds on a cookie sheet and then store it in plastic wrap in the refrigerator. If it's frozen, make sure you place each mound on the prepared dessert at least twenty minutes before serving.

USE FOOD TO SERVE FOOD. Hollowed-out watermelons or pineapples are great for fruit sliced or rounded into balls.

GARNISHES ARE THE STYLISH WOMAN'S ACCESSORIES.
- For yellow garnishes: lemon wedges, summer squash slices.
- For green garnishes: parsley, fresh dill, olives, watercress, green onion tops, zucchini slices.
- For white garnishes: sliced mushrooms (dip in lemon juice to retain color), radishes (white), sliced turnip, egg whites, cauliflower.
- For red garnishes: peppers, pimentos, apples, cranberries, red onions, cherry tomatoes.

PREPARE COFFEE POT (with extension cord if necessary) in advance, but don't perk or drip the coffee.

IF DISASTER STRIKES. The stylish way out . . .
- *The Soufflé Falls or the Jell-O Mold Mushes.* Spoon it into delicate glasses and serve as pudding or parfaits.
- *The Sauce Is Lumpy.* Strain it through a strainer with tiny holes or blend it in a blender.
- *The Pasta Is Nothing More Than Lumps.* Add a little oil and separate the pasta by hand. (TIP: Always buy *semolina* pasta—it's the best!)
- *The Gravy or Stew (or Whatever) Is Too Salty.* Add a peeled potato for a few minutes, which absorbs the salt. Discard the potato.
- *You Drop the Roast on the Way to the Table in Full View of Everyone.* Smile and say, "Fortunately, I've got an identical roast in the kitchen." (Go in the kitchen, rinse off the roast, and serve—after putting fresh parsley on it.)
- *Forget to Put the Wine in the Fridge?* Put it in the freezer for a few minutes.

Dream Dining

I've given you the basics of Party Style. Now let's really get down to business. There can be no party without truly stellar food. What follows are the

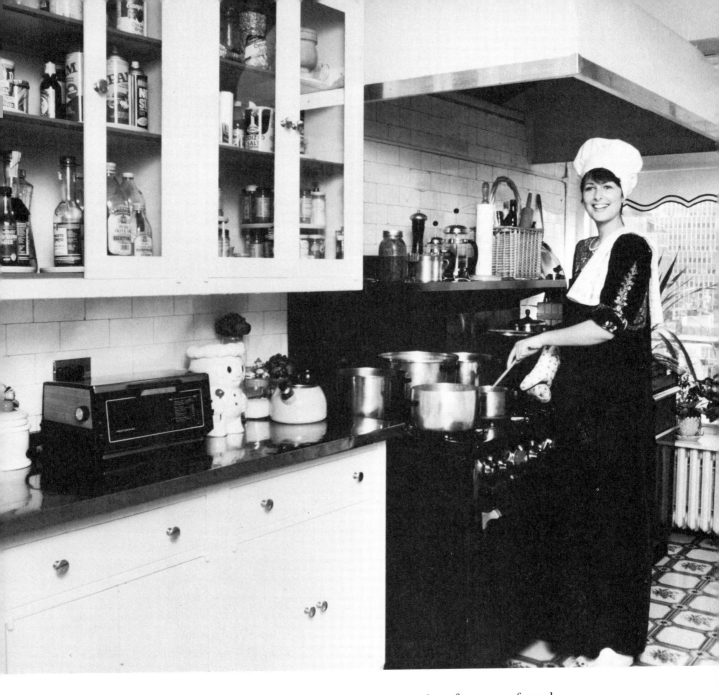

treasure maps to different dining experiences: my own recipes for a very formal dinner party for twelve people *and* the plan for a dinner party on an informal basis for fifty people. And something else. . . .

For years I've been spending a whole lot of money to periodically unwind at an exquisite place called the Golden Door spa. There I exercise, rest, walk, think —and dine royally on the most dazzling cuisine prepared by owner Deborah Szekely's chef, Michael Stroot. I can remember writing down, rather surreptitiously, those treasured recipes I managed to wheedle out of Chef Michael for my family to enjoy, and now, because she's such a wonderful and generous friend,

Deborah has given me permission to reproduce some of my *most* favorite recipes in this book. They are really quite spectacular. Enjoy. Many guests at my parties have whimpered for second helpings.

THE $60 (*Give or Take a Couple of Dollars*)
FORMAL DINNER FOR TWELVE
(*So Elegant You Could Invite Di and Charles*)

During the preparation of this book, I decided to put my money where my mouth was. After *writing* the rules for a formal dinner party . . . I decided to *have* one and asked Roger Prigent, the photographer for this book, to follow me around as I shopped and prepared. My budget was set at sixty dollars, which would not include flowers or liquor. I would serve the most delicious dinner with flowers and candlelight and invite ten friends to share it with John and me—for less than a haircut and body wave in an expensive beauty salon. NOTE: The flowers and wine were later purchased at seventeen dollars, and the dinner's total came to three dollars over budget, which brought a grand total of eighty dollars for *everything!* That amounted to a drop more than six dollars per person. I think that's a great price—considering the gourmet repast and the look of the formal dinner party.

Note from Sherry, the coauthor of this book: "I didn't believe Cristina could pull this dinner party off—not in the style she was accustomed to before the real world plunged her into a budget-conscious mode. *I* could not make an elegant dinner party for twelve for sixty dollars—how in the world could she? But she did. I was a guest at this dinner party, but more important, I was a guest at its creation. I followed her to the butcher, to the wholesale florist, to the grocery store where she carefully picked lettuce and cheese and tomatoes as though she were choosing the jewels for a fabulous necklace. Wherever we went, crowds gathered—she does have one of the most famous faces in town—but she ignored them in her quest for the perfect pepper. She coddled, cajoled, and discussed the merits of her choices and rejections with each storekeeper. She was *serious* about her shopping. Cristina Ferrare is serious about her eating. For two days, I watched her cut, slice, and stir pasta, arrange flowers, mug for the photographer, and, by God, she did it! A formal dinner for twelve for sixty dollars."

First, the Menu!

I love to feed my friends, and planning the menu takes careful thought. There should be something for those who eat meat and for those who do not. It should be satisfying but light—not enough to weigh one down. Since I am Italian, the thrust of the meal would be pasta. Before the meal would come:

THE HORS D'OEUVRES

- I prepare a large plate of *raw vegetables* (crudités), which could include carrots, celery, radishes, Chinese peapods, zucchini, peppers, cucumbers, cherry tomatoes, and whatever else is fresh and crisp in the marketplace the day I shop. I serve crudités with a light dip—perhaps a yogurt dill sauce. I never serve peanuts and other junk that take the edge off the meal to come. I don't even serve *good* serious hors d'oeuvres. Just something light. Next would come:

THE APPETIZER

- *Shrimps with Mustard Dill Sauce* (An alternate appetizer could be cold or hot asparagus with the same sauce).

THE ENTRÉES

- *Crepes Stuffed with Ricotta Cheese and Fresh Herbs;*
- *Crepes Stuffed with Veal, Spinach, and Ricotta.*

THE SALAD

- *Bibb lettuce, watercress, arugula, and lemon dressing with fresh herbs.* I always serve salad after a meal because I feel that its light, crisp taste is refreshing—it kind of cleans the palate after the serious stuff. Serving salad first is the same as serving complicated hors d'oeuvres before a meal—both fill up your guests.

  Incidentally, salads ought to be simple, with a romaine or endive lettuce being far superior to an iceberg lettuce which is not pretty, not high in nutrients, and tasteless, in my book. I often chop up fresh broccoli, cauliflower, and scallions in my salad and serve it with a simple olive oil and lemon dressing (lemon freshens the mouth after dinner), *or*, for a dressing to *die from*, walnut oil with fresh walnuts!

BREAD

- *Hot Italian or French loaves with butter.*

THE CHEESES AND FRUIT

- *A very ripe French Brie;*
- *Slices of buffalo mozzarella cheese and slices of fresh tomato with fresh parsley;*
- *A bowl of fresh fruit* (perhaps apples, pears, or a combination).

THE DESSERT

- *Strawberry-Yogurt Ice with Fresh Strawberries.*

REMEMBER: This will not be one of those cripplingly heavy meals where the guests stagger from the table overladen and slightly ill. On the contrary, although it is quite complete, it is also delicate, varied, pretty, yummy. All of these things. The recipes and the price breakdown follow.

The Hard Stuff

Because liquor consumption varies depending on the guests, I did not include the cost of predinner cocktails in the sixty-dollar dinner for twelve. Certainly if you feel your guests will enjoy them, and you have no religious principles that forbid them, cocktails are a relaxant. I don't drink, but I do offer alcohol to my friends.

JUST ONE CAUTION: If you plan to serve wine at dinner—and that always adds a graceful touch—make it good wine, not that by-the-gallon brew that tastes like alcoholic dishwater. You don't have to spend a fortune for good wine—you can get a bottle of nice (not the *best*, but who's looking?) imported or domestic wine for three or four dollars. Style does not consist of pouring wine from a jug that looks as if it belongs slung over the side of a donkey.

Recipes for the $60 Formal Dinner

SHRIMPS WITH MUSTARD DILL SAUCE

This can be made the morning of the party; it should marinate in the sauce for as long as possible but at *least* two hours.

> 3 pounds boiled shrimp, medium size, deveined and cut in half lengthwise (cutting them in half makes them easier to eat *and* gives more for your money)
> 1 cucumber, peeled, seeded, and chopped for taste and volume
> 4 stalks celery, chopped
> 1 red bell pepper, chopped
> Fresh dill (pinch)
> ½ cup chopped fresh parsley
> ¼ cup chopped fresh chives
> 3 whole lemons (squeeze the juice and set aside)
> ½ cup olive oil
> 3 tablespoons Dijon mustard
> 2–3 teaspoons freshly ground black pepper
> Salt, to taste
> Fresh lettuce leaves
> 1 avocado (optional), chopped

Chop all the vegetables and herbs and set aside. Combine the lemon juice, oil, and mustard in a small bowl and mix until smooth. Combine with the vegetables. Add two or three teaspoons of freshly ground pepper, salt *lightly* to taste, then mix. Pour over the shrimps and refrigerate. Serve over fresh lettuce on a chilled plate with chopped avocado added as garnish, if desired.

NOTE: Shrimp optimally should be bought raw and then deveined and cooked. You can buy shrimp already cooked and cleaned for almost twice the price. Don't! Learn how to do it yourself.

STUFFED CREPES

THE CREPES (About 24)

        1 cup water
        1 cup low-fat milk
        3 eggs
        3 tablespoons melted unsalted butter
        1 teaspoon salt
        2 cups unbleached all-purpose flour
            Small amount of vegetable oil

Put the water, milk, eggs, melted butter and salt in the blender and blend for a few seconds. Add the flour and mix by hand with a spatula (stopping to wipe the sides of the bowl with spatula occasionally). Mix by hand until everything is blended and of a smooth consistency. This mixture should be prepared beforehand and allowed to stand for a couple of hours.

Make the crepes in an eight-inch frying pan using a light vegetable oil to coat the pan. Heat the pan. Add one scant soup ladle of mixture to the middle of the pan and slowly move it around until the bottom of the pan is covered. Cook until you can easily lift the crepe with a spatula and then flip it. Cook the alternate side for five to six seconds or until it easily slides off the pan. Stack the crepes on paper towels.

RICOTTA CHEESE AND FRESH HERB FILLING*

        4½ pounds ricotta cheese
         3 eggs
        ¼ cup freshly grated Parmesan cheese
        ¼ cup freshly grated Romano cheese

* Note for fillings: Each recipe is enough for all twenty-four crepes. If you make half cheese and half veal and spinach, halve the filling recipes.

½ cup chopped fresh parsley
¼ cup chopped fresh chives
1 teaspoon salt
2 teaspoons freshly ground black pepper

Mix the ricotta cheese with the other ingredients. Spoon three helpings of filling onto each crepe, roll, place in a baking dish seam side down, and bake at 350 degrees for forty-five minutes to an hour.

VEAL, SPINACH, AND RICOTTA FILLING

3 pounds ground veal
1–2 tablespoons olive oil
1½ pounds ricotta cheese
2 boxes frozen, chopped spinach, cooked and drained well
2 eggs
½ cup freshly grated Romano cheese
½ cup freshly grated Parmesan cheese
1 teaspoon nutmeg
Salt and freshly ground black pepper, to taste
Béchamel sauce (See below.)

Place the veal in a frying pan with one or two tablespoons of olive oil. Cook the meat slowly until done (do *not* fry). When it has cooled, place it in a large bowl and add the ricotta cheese. Mix well. Add the spinach, eggs, and other cheeses. Mix well. Add the nutmeg, salt, and pepper. Pour the béchamel sauce over the mixture and stir. Spoon three heaping tablespoons into each crepe and roll. You may cut the crepes in half at this point, which makes them easier to serve. Place in large baking pan, neatly, seam side down. Bake at 350 degrees for forty-five minutes to an hour.

BÉCHAMEL SAUCE

3 tablespoons unsalted butter
3 tablespoons unbleached, all-purpose flour
1 cup warm whole milk
1 teaspoon salt

Melt the butter, add the flour, and mix until lumpy. Slowly add the milk and stir with a wire whisk until the mixture is smoothly blended. Cook over a low heat until it becomes thickened and smooth, stirring continuously.

SAUCE FOR CREPES—TOMATO CONCASSEE

I often use this Golden Door recipe to spoon over the crepes.

- 4 teaspoons olive oil
- 2 garlic cloves, chopped
- 2 tablespoons minced shallots
- 2 tablespoons dried sweet basil
- 2 bay leaves
- 10 large tomatoes, peeled and finely diced (or 2 18-ounce cans whole plum tomatoes)
- 2 teaspoons freshly ground black pepper

Gently sauté the garlic and shallots in oil. Add the basil, bay leaves, tomatoes, and pepper. Cover and simmer for five minutes. Then simmer uncovered for ten to fifteen minutes more. (You can make this sauce in advance and freeze it.)

STRAWBERRY-YOGURT ICE WITH FRESH STRAWBERRIES

- 2 quarts strawberry ice cream
- 2 cups low-fat plain yogurt
- 3 cups sliced strawberries
- Whole strawberries for garnish

Purée everything together in a blender until quite smooth. Pour into glasses that will not crack in the freezer. Chill in the freezer for two hours, then refrigerate for about half an hour. Serve with extra fresh strawberries (or sliced kiwi fruit). (For a bit of extra elegance, you can pour a bit of bubbly champagne over each dessert right at the table.)

THE $60 FORMAL-DINNER PRICE BREAKDOWN

Hors d'Oeuvres (Crudités)—Approximately $4.00
Shrimps with Mustard Dill Sauce—Approximately $21.00
Crepes with two different fillings—Approximately $17.00
Dessert—$7.00
Bread—$3.00
Cheese and fruit—$6.00
Salad—$5.00

Total: $63.00

THE $150 INFORMAL BUFFET FOR FIFTY PEOPLE

If I don't have help or a very minimum of help, I often prefer a buffet type of dinner where every dish can be set out on a large table and people help themselves. Tables can range from a preset table to stack tables to the floor. If the choice is stack tables or the floor, be sure to serve food that doesn't require complicated cutting, like crepes, fish, pasta, or casserole-type stews. Sometimes help-yourself buffets are combined with a served dessert. You can economize on types of wine and flowers; you can bake rather than buy, but *never* cook too little —that's really embarrassing. If there's food left over, you can freeze it or, for goodwill credit, send some home with your helper. An informal buffet is a perfect time to throw a really *large* party. What follows are the recipes for a buffet dinner I made for my friend's birthday party. It cost me $150 (not including wine and flowers) and fifty people were invited! Three dollars per head!! Better than that you *Cannot* do.

Menu for a $150 Buffet for Fifty

Have to throw a big party for a whole lot of people? It can be done—simply, elegantly, and inexpensively. What's more, the buffet table will include food for meat eaters, dieters, and vegetarians, so no one—God forbid—has to go home hungry. Here's what's on your table:

ON ONE SIDE OF THE TABLE
- *A huge vegetarian salad*—Include things like mixed greens (watercress, romaine, Boston lettuce, and so on), avocado, sliced carrots and peppers, cucumber, scallions, artichoke hearts, alfalfa sprouts, raw sliced mushrooms . . . use your imagination!
- *A plate of sliced tomatoes alternating with sliced buffalo mozzarella cheese and fresh basil.* A good dressing for both the salad and the tomato plate is the mustard vinaigrette found on page 199.
- *A large fruit salad.* Perhaps, in a scooped-out watermelon as container, include honeydew, cantaloupe, strawberries, kiwi fruit, grapefruit, orange slices, raspberries, peaches . . . whatever's in season.

continued on next page

IN THE CENTER OF THE TABLE
- *A large Poached Salmon surrounded by Salmon Mousse.*
- *A Cucumber Marinade with Green Dill Sauce.*
- *Chicken Piccata* (Boneless, skinless chicken—low in calories and delicious).

ON THE OTHER SIDE OF THE TABLE
- *Stuffed Pasta Shells* (Some with meat, spinach and ricotta; others just with ricotta for vegetarians).

DESSERT, BUFFET STYLE
- *Many balls of assorted ice creams* put in your finest crystal bowls; dishes of toppings and walnuts (optional); hot fudge, coconut, butterscotch.
- *Coffee and tea.*

Recipes for the Informal Buffet

POACHED SALMON

10-12	pounds raw salmon (in one piece), cleaned
4	tablespoons unsalted butter
½	cup chopped celery
½	cup chopped carrot
½	cup chopped onion
	Enough cold water to cover fish
1	cup dry white wine
4–6	whole peppercorns
	Lemon slices and fresh dill for garnish

Melt the butter in large skillet, add the chopped vegetables, and cook gently for five minutes. Add water, wine, and pepper and cook for five minutes more. Wrap the salmon in a large piece of cheesecloth and place it on a rack that fits in the skillet (or use fish poacher). The water mixture should cover the fish. Place the skillet on top of stove and simmer very gently for one to one and a half hours, depending on the size of the fish. (Figure about eight minutes to a pound: Fish is done when it flakes easily.) Remove it from the pan, drain it carefully, and gently remove the cheesecloth. Serve it on a pretty tray garnished with wafer-thin slices of lemon and sprinklings of fresh dill.

SALMON MOUSSE

4 pound poached salmon (as in previous recipe)
1 cup heavy cream
2 cups mayonnaise
1 teaspoon chopped fresh dill
1 tablespoon chopped fresh chives
4 tablespoons minced scallions
2 tablespoons grainy mustard
1½ tablespoons salt and a sprinkling of freshly ground black pepper
2 envelopes unflavored gelatin
Fish broth (amount needed for gelatin)

Bone and flake the poached fish and blend with the other ingredients in a blender or food processor set on low speed. Dissolve the gelatin according to the directions, but use fish broth instead of water. Fold it into the mixture. Oil one large or two small fish-shaped molds and scoop the salmon mixture into mold. Refrigerate for at least four hours before serving.

CUCUMBER MARINADE WITH GREEN DILL SAUCE

20 large cucumbers
8 tablespoons Dijon mustard
Juice of 4 lemons
2 cups olive oil
4 teaspoons fresh, cracked peppercorns
16 tablespoons chopped fresh dill

Peel the cucumbers. Put them through a food processor if possible; if not, simply chop them very finely. Mix the mustard, lemon juice, and olive oil with spoon until blended (do not put in a blender). Stir this mixture into the chopped cucumbers. Add the pepper and dill and mix gently. Refrigerate at least an hour before serving.

CHICKEN PICCATA

32 chicken breasts (ask your butcher to bone and skin them
   —*and* flatten them out)
4 cups sifted unbleached, all-purpose flour
2½ cups olive oil
16 cloves garlic, mashed
   Juice of 16 lemons
4 cups sherry (not cooking wine—the real stuff)
½ cup chopped parsley
½ cup capers (optional)

Cut the chicken into bite-sized portions. Dip them lightly into the flour
and sauté them in olive oil with the garlic until they are brown. Add the
lemon juice and sherry and cook covered on a low heat for ten to fifteen
minutes. Serve in a casserole dish with fresh parsley and, if desired,
capers sprinkled on top.

PASTA SHELLS STUFFED WITH RICOTTA CHEESE

10 pounds pasta shells (That's more than you need, but it
   will give you extra for those that break—and they will!
   The best place to buy pasta shells is in an Italian
   delicatessen, although every supermarket carries
   them.)
15 pounds ricotta cheese
4 pounds freshly grated Parmesan cheese
4 cups fresh, chopped parsley
5½ tablespoons freshly ground black pepper
12 whole eggs, lightly beaten
2½ teaspoons salt (optional)
   Butter to grease baking dish

Boil the pasta, al dente, according to the package directions. Cool
slightly. Mix the ricotta cheese with 2 pounds of the grated Parmesan
cheese and other ingredients. Stuff the shells with the mixture. Place
the stuffed shells in a greased baking dish, pour the tomato sauce (recipe
follows) on top, and sprinkle the remainder of grated Parmesan cheese
on top of that. Cover with aluminum foil. Bake in a preheated 350 degree
oven for about a half hour. During the last five minutes, remove the
cover. Serve bubbly and hot in chafing dish.

TOMATO SAUCE

1 medium onion
1 medium carrot
1 stalk celery
2 cloves garlic
2 ounces salt pork
⅓ cup olive oil
2 cans (1 pound) Italian plum tomatoes
  Salt and freshly ground pepper to taste

Place the onion, carrot, celery, garlic and salt pork in a food processor and chop coarsely. Sauté in olive oil until the onion is transparent. Chop the canned tomatoes in food processor, then add to the sautéed ingredients. Simmer, uncovered, on very low heat for about one and a half hours until the sauce reaches a thick, rich consistency. Stir in the salt and pepper to taste and serve.

GOLDEN DOOR CUISINE

TAKE YOUR CHOICE FROM

Two vegetable dishes;
Two salads;
Two fowl dishes;
One fish dish;
One meat dish;
One side dish;
Two fabulous desserts.

VEGETABLE DISHES

BROCCOLI SOUFFLÉ

10 ounces broccoli tops, cut in chunks
1½ cups water
2½ tablespoons corn oil margarine
3½ tablespoons unbleached, all-purpose flour
½ teaspoon dried sweet basil
  Grated nutmeg, to taste

¼ teaspoon white pepper
   ¼ teaspoon vegetable seasoning
   4 tablespoons grated Parmesan or Romano cheese
   3 egg yolks
   2 teaspoons low-fat milk
   5 egg whites, room temperature
     Sea salt
     Cream of tartar

In a covered saucepan, gently cook the broccoli tops, covered with water, until they are tender (about fifteen minutes). Drain the broccoli. Reserve 1 cup of the broth. Chop the broccoli finely or use a food processor.

Over a low fire, melt the margarine and add the flour, stirring with a wire whisk to make a paste (roux). Pour the broccoli broth into the roux and whisk vigorously until the mixture becomes a thick sauce and bubbles. Add the basil, nutmeg, pepper, vegetable seasoning, three tablespoons of the grated cheese, and the chopped broccoli. Cook three to four minutes. Remove the mixture from the stove, and transfer it to a bowl. Stir occasionally to cool. When cooled, beat the egg yolks with the milk, and stir it into the mixture. (This can be prepared several hours in advance.)

Preheat oven to 350 degrees. Beat the egg whites with a pinch of salt and a pinch of cream of tartar until they are stiff. Fold one-quarter of the whites into the broccoli mixture. Gently fold in the remainder. Pour the mixture into four lightly oiled one-and-three-quarter-cup souf-flé dishes. Sprinkle each with the remaining cheese. Place the soufflé dishes on a baking tray. Bake for twenty minutes. Reduce the heat to 325 degrees, and bake fifteen minutes more. Serve immediately. This makes four soufflés at 233 calories per serving. Preparation time is thirty-five minutes, and baking time is thirty to thirty-five minutes.

ZUCCHINI-SPINACH FRITTATA

   3 cups grated zucchini
   1 tablespoon vegetable seasoning
   ¾ cup cooked fresh spinach, squeezed and chopped
   1 teaspoon dried sweet basil
   1 tablespoon freshly grated Parmesan or Romano cheese
   ½ teaspoon freshly ground black pepper
   2 tablespoons coarsely chopped chives or green onions
   4 whole eggs
   2 egg whites
   ¼ cup low-fat milk

        2 teaspoons minced garlic
        1 medium onion, diced
        1 teaspoon dried whole thyme
        2 teaspoons olive oil
        1 cup thickly sliced raw mushrooms
        ½ cup thickly sliced artichoke hearts
        3 ounces mozzarella cheese, sliced

Preheat the oven to 350 degrees. In a large bowl, grate the zucchini and add the vegetable seasoning. Mix well. Put in a colander and let stand about a half-hour. Combine with the chopped spinach. Add the basil, cheese, pepper, and chives. Mix well.

In separate bowl, beat the whole eggs, egg whites, and milk. Combine with zucchini mixture. In a nine-inch skillet, gently sauté the garlic, onion, and thyme in oil until they start to soften. Add the mushrooms; stir with a wooden spoon until they start to soften. Add the artichokes and heat well.

Transfer the mixture to a casserole dish. Pour the spinach/zucchini mixture over the onion mixture. Let this bubble for a few seconds. Cover with the sliced cheese. Bake for forty to forty-five minutes, or until a knife comes out clean when inserted in the center. Remove from the oven and let sit for ten minutes before serving. Serve with Tomato Concassee sauce (page 191).

This makes eight small portions at 111 calories per portion or four large portions at 222 calories per portion. Preparation time is one hour, thirty-five minutes.

SALADS

TOMATO OREGANO

        4 tomatoes, peeled
        1 tablespoon chopped shallots
        1 teaspoon minced garlic
        1 teaspoon dried whole oregano (or 4 fresh basil leaves)
        3 tablespoons Mustard Vinaigrette Dressing (see below)
        3 teaspoons chives
          Lettuce leaves to line 4 plates

Cut each tomato into eight wedges. Put into salad bowl. Add the shallots, garlic, and oregano (or basil leaves). Spoon on Mustard Vinaigrette Dressing and mix well. Refrigerate for four hours.

Spoon onto four lettuce beds, sprinkle on chives and serve. This serves four at 77 calories per serving. Preparation time is fifteen minutes.

MUSTARD VINAIGRETTE DRESSING

> 1 tablespoon Dijon mustard
> 1 teaspoon freshly ground black pepper
> 5½ tablespoons apple-cider vinegar
> 6½ tablespoons sesame seed or safflower oil
> 1 tablespoon water

Mix together all ingredients in an eight-ounce jar. Before using, close the lid tightly and shake vigorously. This is a strong dressing and should be used sparingly. It is excellent with a green bean–tomato salad, crudités, and other salads.

NOTE: This keeps well under refrigeration.

Each tablespoon has 59 calories. Preparation time is five minutes.

CALIFORNIA-STYLE SALAD

Mixed greens (romaine, Boston lettuce, watercress, spinach, etc.) to make 4 portions

> 4 tablespoons Lemon Dressing (see below)
> 3 tablespoons sesame seeds, freshly toasted
> 12 large grapefruit wedges
> 1 ripe avocado, peeled and thinly sliced
> 1 Bermuda onion, thinly sliced and marinated in vinegar
>   Parsley sprigs for garnish

Toss the salad greens with the Lemon Dressing and sesame seeds. Place in four chilled bowls. On each salad, place three grapefruit wedges alternated with three avocado slices; top with two or three onion rings.

Garnish with parsley and serve. This serves four at 233 calories per serving. Preparation time is fifteen minutes.

LEMON DRESSING

> 4 tablespoons sesame seed or safflower oil
> 3 tablespoons fresh lemon juice
> 2 tablespoons chopped fresh parsley
> ½ teaspoon vegetable seasoning
> ¼ teaspoon freshly ground black pepper
> 2–3 tablespoons freshly grated Parmesan or Romano cheese

Place all ingredients except the cheese in a blender. Blend until the parsley is finely chopped. Add the cheese when tossing the salad.

NOTE: To preserve the fresh lemon flavor, prepare this dressing just before serving.

This makes three-quarters of a cup of dressing at 96 calories per tablespoon. Preparation time is five minutes.

FOWL

BROILED CORNISH GAME HEN GOLDEN DOOR

    2 Cornish game hens (1 pound, 5 ounces each), halved
    2 tablespoons soy sauce (low sodium)
    1 teaspoon minced fresh ginger
    ⅓ cup pineapple juice
    8 thin orange slices, seeded
    2 teaspoons coconut, grated and freshly toasted
      Parsley sprigs for garnish

Cover and refrigerate game hens in a marinade of the soy sauce, ginger, and pineapple juice for two hours.

Preheat the broiler. Remove the hens from marinade, setting marinade aside. Place the hens in a skillet; broil five minutes on each side. Remove and preheat oven to 350 degrees. Bake the hens in the oven, uncovered, for thirty minutes, until done. In the same skillet, pour the marinade over the hens and mix it with pan juices. Simmer the hens on top of the stove for two to three minutes to reduce the juice.

Serve hens in their juice topped with orange slices and coconut sprinkle. Garnish with parsley and serve. This serves four at 285 calories per serving. Preparation time is forty-five minutes.

SESAME CHICKEN BREAST IN GINGER

    2 whole chicken breasts cut in half, skinned, boned, and trimmed of fat
    1 tablespoon minced fresh ginger
    1 tablespoon soy sauce (low sodium)
    2 tablespoons sesame seed or safflower oil
    4 teaspoons minced garlic
    1 cup fresh asparagus, trimmed, cut into pieces 2 inches long
    1 cup zucchini, cut into pieces 2 inches long

1 cup scallions (green part), cut into pieces 2 inches long
½ cup chicken broth, heated
3 cups bean sprouts
   Soy sauce (low sodium)
   Vegetable seasoning
1 tablespoon arrowroot (dissolved in 2 tablespoons water)
1 teaspoon grated lemon zest (yellow part of rind)
3 tablespoons sesame seeds, freshly toasted

Marinate chicken breasts in the ginger and mild soy sauce for one hour. Cut the chicken breasts into thin strips two inches long. In a heavy skillet, quickly heat one tablespoon oil and two teaspoons garlic. Stir in the chicken strips until they are lightly sautéed.

Cover, remove from heat, and set aside. Use a wok to stir-fry the vegetables: Heat the remainder of the oil and garlic, and in quick succession add the asparagus and zucchini. Stir-fry until the vegetables begin to cook. Add the chicken strips and scallions; mix again. Add the chicken broth and bean sprouts; sprinkle with soy sauce and vegetable seasoning. When the broth comes to a boil, thicken with dissolved arrowroot. The whole process should take about ten minutes.

Before serving, sprinkle with lemon zest and sesame seeds. This serves four at 274 calories per serving. It can be prepared one hour in advance. Cooking time is fifteen minutes.

FISH

BAKED DILL SALMON

1 pound salmon fillets, cut into four portions
12 ⅛-inch-thick cucumber slices, peeled
4 lemon slices, peeled
1 teaspoon dried dill
4 parsley sprigs
4 large raw shrimp (optional), peeled and deveined

This may be baked or barbecued. If baked, preheat the oven to 375 degrees. Place the salmon on twelve-inch-square pieces of foil. Spread three cucumber slices and one lemon slice on each fish portion. Sprinkle with dill; add one parsley sprig and, if desired, one shrimp. Lift the ends of the foil and close them tightly together to make a pouch.

Put the salmon about three to four inches above the hot fire of a barbecue grill, a little away from center of heat. Cook fifteen to twenty minutes. Or put the foil-wrapped salmon in a baking dish and bake in the oven for twenty minutes, or until done. Remove the fish from the foil and serve immediately with salad and crudités.

This serves four at 156 calories per serving. Preparation time is thirty minutes.

MEAT

VEAL SCALOPPINE

> 4 veal scaloppine (white veal—2½–3 ounces each)
> Unbleached, all-purpose white flour, to dust
> 1 egg, beaten
> 2 teaspoons dried whole oregano
> 2 tablespoons freshly grated Parmesan cheese
> 1 tablespoon olive oil
> 2 tablespoons unsalted butter or corn oil margarine
> 1 tablespoon minced chives or scallions
> 1 cup diced, cooked artichoke hearts (fresh or canned)
> 2 cups sliced fresh mushrooms
> ½ teaspoon freshly ground black pepper
> ½ cup dry white wine
> ½ cup chicken broth, heated
> ¼ cup fresh lemon juice
> 4 tablespoons freshly chopped parsley

Preheat the oven to 350 degrees. To the beaten egg, add one teaspoon oregano and one tablespoon cheese. Quickly dust the scaloppine in flour and dip in the egg wash.

In large heavy skillet over a low fire, heat the olive oil and quickly sauté the scaloppine for two minutes on each side, until golden brown. Place it in a baking dish, cover loosely with foil, and set in the oven for no more than ten minutes while preparing the sauce.

In same skillet heat one tablespoon of butter and sauté the chives or scallions. Add the remaining one teaspoon of oregano and cook briefly. Add the artichokes and mushrooms and stir with wooden spatula until mushrooms begin to cook. Sprinkle with pepper. Pour over the wine, chicken broth, and lemon juice. Reduce the heat for three to four minutes, and add the remaining butter.

Remove the scaloppine from the oven; place it in the skillet to soak up the sauce. Sprinkle with the remaining cheese and with parsley. Serve immediately.

Accompany this dish with peeled and sliced Jerusalem artichokes and plain spaghetti with perhaps a little butter and fresh parsley spooned into it. This serves four at 240 calories per serving. Preparation time is one hour.

SIDE DISH

GOLDEN POTATO SKINS

    4 large baking potatoes
    1 tablespoon sesame seed or safflower oil
    1 teaspoon vegetable seasoning

Preheat the oven to 375 degrees. Wash and scrub the potatoes. Rub with a little oil. Bake for about one hour and fifteen minutes, until done. Remove the potatoes from the oven, place a damp towel over them (prevents the skins from drying out), and cool. This step can be prepared several hours in advance.

    Again preheat the oven to 375 degrees. Halve the cooled potatoes lengthwise. Scoop out the insides, and set aside. (Leave about a half inch of potato next to the skin.) Season the skins with vegetable seasoning and brush lightly with oil. Bake thirty minutes longer, until they are crisp and lightly browned. Serve immediately. This serves four at 40 calories per serving. Preparation time is fifteen minutes, and baking time is one hour, forty-five minutes.

DESSERTS

HOT BANANAS AND BLUEBERRIES

    4 ripe bananas
    ⅓ cup apple juice (unfiltered)
    ½ cup fresh blueberries (or 2 teaspoons candied ginger)
    1 tablespoon Cointreau or Grand Marnier orange liqueur
      Mint sprigs, strawberries, or kiwi slices for garnish

Place the bananas in skillet with the apple juice. Simmer gently, covered, for four to five minutes, until the bananas start to soften. Turn the bananas over. Cook, uncovered, for three to four minutes longer, to reduce liquid to half. Add the berries or ginger.

    Remove from heat. Add the liqueur. Shake the skillet to roll the bananas in the liquid. Serve immediately with its juice, garnished. This makes eight small portions at 60 calories per portion or four large portions at 120 calories per portion. Preparation time is ten minutes.

PEARS IN BURGUNDY WINE AND CASSIS

        2 tablespoons sun-dried currants
        2 tablespoons Creme de Cassis liqueur
        ¾ cup plus 2 tablespoons Burgundy wine
        ½ cup water
        1 tablespoon fresh lemon juice
        1 tablespoon honey
        2 cloves
        1 large, ripe pear, halved lengthwise and cored
          Mint sprigs and lemon slices for garnish

Soak the currants in the Cassis liqueur and two tablespoons of Burgundy for about an hour.

Bring to a boil the three-quarters of a cup of Burgundy, the water, lemon juice, honey, and cloves. Simmer for five minutes. Drop in the pear halves and gently poach, uncovered, for ten minutes, until tender but still a little firm. Remove the pears with a slotted spoon. Reduce the liquid by one-third. Remove from heat; add the currants.

Cool the liquid and pour it over pears. Chill. Garnish and serve. This recipe can be prepared a day in advance. It serves four at 163 calories per serving. Preparation time is twenty minutes.

Epilogue

PICTURE a chic room with sparkling conversation, elegant furniture, and familiar faces. Picture the buzz of busy, passionate, laughing voices. And then picture the room growing suddenly silent for just a minute.

A woman of style has quietly come into the picture.

It's not that she's exquisite. It's that she's unflappable. Cool. In control. You just have to look at her.

You'd know her anywhere because her style lies in the way she holds her head, orders in a restaurant, talks with warmth and concern to the grocer. Her style is the illusion of perfect features, wealth, and wit—even though she may have none of these. Her style is glamour. Paying attention to detail.

Some people seem to be born with that attitude of self-assurance, that ability to create presence. They bring panache to the most unlikely places—the supermarket, the word processor room, the kitchen. Others have carefully acquired their style, and that's even better than being born with it.

Although money certainly helps, it is by no means the only road to style. In fact, some people are distinctly uncomfortable with money. They don't know how to deal with it. There are as many people who apologize for being rich as for being poor. Both are graceless acts. Perhaps the greatest spokesman for style in poverty *and* wealth is that brilliantly irreverent stylist Quentin Crisp, who makes his living just being Quentin Crisp, "If you haven't got anything, flaunt it," says Crisp. On the other hand, he adds, "You must never feel guilty about being rich . . . and don't go around carrying your own garment bag (like Jimmy Carter) to try to show that you're 'regular folks.' " The important thing, says Crisp, is to understand that "it is as foolish to base your style on your money as it is to base it on your beauty or your job, for if you ever lose your money (or your beauty or your job), you lose your style along with it." If anyone knows that's true, it's me. Style in the real world transcends rich *and* poor. Which is why, I suppose, my best friend, Eileen, made me a pillow that says "Nouveau Is Better Than Not Riche at All." Naturally I believe that with all my heart.

I like to think that a woman of style is a happy mixture between old and new money and between poverty and upward mobility. You can never, in other words, put a price tag on style. It used to be a Fifth Avenue duplex and a DeLorean automobile, among other things, in my world. Now it's mostly my frame of mind. *Positive*, if you will.

Anyone, I truly believe, can learn to be the woman for whom the room quiets as she enters.